Review of Research in Nursing Education Volume VI

Review of Research in Nursing Education Volume VI

Lois Ryan Allen, PhD, RN
Editor

National League for Nursing • New York
Pub. No. 19-2544

ISBN 0-88737-596-0

The views expressed in this publication represent the views of the authors and do not necessarily reflect the official views of the National League for Nursing.

This book was set in Baskerville by Publications Development Company. The editor and designer was Allan Graubard. Automated Graphic Systems was the printer and binder.

Printed in the United States of America

EDITORIAL REVIEW BOARD

CONTRIBUTORS

Barbra Bachmeier, BSN, RN
Graduate Student
Indiana University School of Nursing
Indianapolis, Indiana

Diane M. Billings, EdD, RN, FAAN
Professor of Nursing
Assistant Dean of Learning Resources
Indiana University School of Nursing
Indianapolis, Indiana

Dona Marie Carpenter, EdD, RN
Assistant Professor of Nursing
University of Scranton
Scranton, Pennsylvania

Betsy Frank, PhD, RN
Visiting Assistant Professor
University of New Mexico College of Nursing
Albuquerque, New Mexico

Sharon Hudacek, EdD, RN
Assistant Professor of Nursing
University of Scranton
Scranton, Pennsylvania

Janice M. Layton, PhD, RN
Professor and Chairperson
Department of Nursing
California State University
San Bernardino, California

Bonnie L. Saucier, PhD, RN
Professor and Chairperson
Department of Nursing
California State University
Bakersfield, California

PREFACE

The NLN Council for Research in Nursing Education (CRNE) is pleased to present Volume VI of the Review of Research in Nursing Education series. Publication of the Review series is one way in which the CRNE facilitates the dissemination of nursing education research findings. Each Review chapter presents an analysis of the research literature in a specific area. The chapters in Volume VI address pertinent topics for nursing education and nursing education research as the CRNE moves forward into its second decade. Empathy and caring, two identified outcomes of the recent curriculum revolution, are addressed in chapters by Layton and Frank. Billings and Bachmeier review the literature on distance education and Saucier explores the issue of student retention. Both of these topics are of critical concern in nursing education today, given the changing demographics of the current student population. Hudacek and Carpenter review the development of doctoral programs in nursing education, with attention to the similarities and differences among programs. Each chapter concludes with the authors' thought-provoking questions or ideas about new directions for future research.

Each chapter was peer reviewed by at least two members of the Editorial Board. As Editor of this volume, I want to express my sincere appreciation to the members of the Editorial Board for their time, effort, and expertise. All inquiries, letters of interest, or outlines for future chapter submissions should be directed to:

Kathleen Stevens, EdD, RN
Associate Professor
School of Nursing
University of Texas Health Science Center
San Antonio, TX 78284

CONTENTS

Chapter One

TEACHING AND LEARNING AT A DISTANCE: A REVIEW OF THE NURSING LITERATURE

Diane M. Billings, EdD, RN, FAAN
Barbra Bachmeier, BSN, RN

INTRODUCTION

As increasing numbers of nurses and nursing students seek access to education and live at a distance from institutions offering basic and continuing education, schools of nursing and health care agencies are restructuring instructional systems to establish learning communities that are both accessible and cost-effective. At the same time, the instructional technologies available via television and computers are becoming increasingly accessible and their costs are decreasing. The purpose of this review is to examine critically the nursing literature regarding distance education in order to assist nurse educators and administrators in making informed decisions about the use and effectiveness of distance education. Recommendations for additional research in the field follow.

DISTANCE EDUCATION IN NURSING

Distance education, the separation of teacher and student during study, uses print and electronic media for connecting people who have learning needs to resources to meet those needs. With distance education, there is a "virtual classroom" that transcends limitations of time and space. Distance education emphasizes the design of instruction, support of the learner, interaction between the student and faculty, and evaluation of learning outcomes. Thus, for lessons, modules, courses, or entire nursing degree programs, there is a seamless system of instruction that can be delivered where the learner is—at home, worksite, community learning center, or institution of higher education.

Distance education involves both teaching and learning. Distance *teaching* focuses on the role of the institution and faculty in offering the course or program; distance *learning* focuses on the student and student support (Clarke & Cohen, 1992). Distance *education* involves the interaction among the delivery system (medium), management and administration of the instruction, instructional support, and evaluation of these components (Heath, 1991).

DISTANCE EDUCATION DELIVERY SYSTEMS

Distance education uses a variety of media to support instructional communication. These include print, audio, television, and the computer. Often, two or more media are used to maximize benefits and offset limitations inherent in each delivery system.

Print-Based Delivery Systems

Distance education using print media occurs through paper-and-pencil exchanges between student and faculty. *Correspondence* instruction (Billings, 1987; Billings, Marriner, & Smith, 1986) is a series of self-contained, preplanned, preproduced lessons conducted by noncontiguous communication, usually via mail or fax. Correspondence courses offer lessons and examinations, with student faculty interaction occurring through lesson feedback and evaluation. Correspondence courses are typically offered for credit and managed by an independent study division of a college or university.

Self-paced (self-directed or self-instructional) learning, like correspondence courses, involves self-contained, print-based instructional units, but focuses on one topic (Chick & Paull, 1988; Rufo, 1985) and is not transmitted through the mail. These lessons/programs/learning packages/modules contain pre-/posttests, objectives, exercises, study guides, assignments, learning activities, and, possibly, a clinical component (Rufo, 1985). There is emphasis on the learner, who assumes responsibility for initiating, completing, and evaluating the learning experiences (Brunt & Scott, 1986; DeSilets, 1986; Haggard, 1992; Hamilton & Gregor, 1986; Hast, 1987; Huckaby, 1981; Wiley, 1983). In *self-directed* learning, the faculty supports, guides, and provides feedback. A contract can be used to facilitate lesson completion. In *self-managed* instruction, lessons are designed like programmed instruction (Goldrick, Appling-Stevens, & Larson, 1990), but, unlike self-paced learning, they do not have the full range of assignments and varying learning activities. *Independent study* (Lethbridge, 1988; Luchsinger, 1990) gives learners control over their learning environment and pace.

Audio-Based Delivery Systems

Instruction can also be delivered using voice and audio technology. *Audioteleconferences* (teleconferences, audioconferences) involve delivering two-way instruction over telephone lines to distant reception sites where students communicate using speaker phones (Guillemin, 1986; Henry, 1993; Kuramoto, 1984; Muse, 1984; Wuest, 1989). Audioconferences decrease isolation, increase student confidence in participating in the distant class, and allow for immediate feedback from participating students (Thompson & Taylor, 1991). When used over dedicated telephone lines, audio-based systems are a cost-effective method to overcome geographic distances. Audioconferences are often used as an adjunct to print-based systems for promoting interactive dialogue with faculty and peers. *Audiographics* (Luchsinger, 1990) uses computer graphics to supplement the audioconference by providing visual support for audioconferences. Although not reported in nursing literature reviewed here, *audiotapes* and *radio* are other examples of audio-based technologies.

Voice mail is a telephone-based computerized messaging system in which digitized voice messages are stored and retrieved by individual students (Bernard & Naidu, 1990). There are "bulletin board" functions, in which instructional "messages" are retrieved by all participants, as well as facilities for messages or instruction for individual students. Although not yet implemented, a needs assessment conducted by Bernard and Naidu (1990) indicated a positive response by nursing students who identified a need for communicating more directly with faculty and classmates.

Video-Based Delivery Systems

Video-based systems use television for instruction by cable, microwave, or satellite on closed or open circuits. *Teleconferencing (videoteleconferencing, videoconferencing, interactive video)* (Billings, Frazier, Lausch, & McCarty, 1989; Boyd & Baker, 1987; Colbert, 1984; Limón, Spencer, & Henderson, 1985; Major & Shane, 1991; Tribulski & Frank, 1987) uses live broadcasts in which the video transmission may be two-way video (reception site and broadcast site see and hear each other), or one-way video and two-way audio (reception site views on a monitor what is transmitted and participates using a microphone through telephone lines). *Video-enhanced teleconferencing* (Kerr, 1988) uses computers and modems to transmit graphics, data, and voice over a telephone line to support instruction.

Unlike videoconferencing, *telecourses* (Clark, 1989) involve videotapes of classes saved for later viewing or shown in health care agencies or students' homes. Because the capabilities of real-time interaction are lost, telecourses are usually accompanied by self-contained syllabi with objectives, learning activities, and examinations (Clark, 1989). *Videotapes* may be used with other print materials, as independent study offerings, or as file tapes of interactive classes, for later use.

Computer-Based Delivery Systems

Instruction can be delivered by computers, using worldwide computer networks (Billings, 1992; Thiele & Higgs, 1992). *Computer conferencing* allows a discussion group to "meet" on an electronic mail system that is part of a computer network. Instruction occurs through the use of a "bulletin board": general information is posted and discussed, but, unlike electronic mail, the students can add their own comments, thus creating opportunities for peer and faculty interaction; communication between individuals is also possible.

THE REVIEW OF LITERATURE

The Search

Using key words—*audioconferencing, audiovisual, correspondence, distance education, independent study, interactive TV, nontraditional education, self-directed learning, self-learning, self-modular learning, teaching methods, telecommunications,* and *teleconference*—nursing (CINAHL) and education (ERIC, CARL) databases from 1966 to 1992 were searched for articles regarding distance education in nursing. Additional sources were revealed in references in these articles. Sixty-nine articles were located and used in this review. Articles about "off-campus" or "satellite" programs were excluded because they do not use print or electronic media to connect learners and teachers, and therefore do not meet the definition of distance education used in this review. Although the search focused on 28 research-based articles in distance education (see Table 1, pp. 6–13), the other articles contributing to the understanding of distance education in nursing were reviewed and included to amplify and clarify the research-based reports. Finally, findings of the research-based articles were categorized into common themes using content analysis procedures.

General Comments and Critique

Of the 28 research-based articles in this review, eleven report on television-based instruction, eight on print-based instruction, two on audio delivery systems, two on computer conferencing, and five on a mix of delivery systems. Six articles describe distance education in countries other than the United States—Canada, Great Britain, Australia, and New Zealand; two articles describe international experiences with distance education. Courses, programs, and continuing education opportunities are offered by distance education to LPN, ADN, BSN, and MSN students for basic and continuing nursing education. Needs surveys (Phillips, Hagenbuch, & Baldwin, 1992; Scheele, Smith, & Perry, 1992) indicate nurses are willing to participate in distance education and may prefer it to other delivery systems. Pym (1992), however, suggests that distance education may not be the nurses' *first* choice for receiving instruction, but is chosen because it permits education for women who have other responsibilities for employment and child care.

The research in distance education is in foundational stages. The studies reviewed here are, by and large, descriptive and evaluative and not guided by theoretical frameworks. Additionally, there is little evidence of using findings from previous studies to extend the knowledge base. Sample sizes tend to be smaller and based on the experiences of faculty and students in one course or module. Lack of clarity in defining instructional delivery systems and instructional settings hinders understanding of what delivery system is being used where, thus making generalizations about the attributes of and relationships between delivery systems and outcomes difficult. Finally, most instruments used in research (primarily surveys) do not have validity and reliability reported and have not been used as a basis for further studies.

A content analysis of the research literature revealed six themes. These are categorized as

1. Advantages and benefits of distance education (access, recruitment and retention, cost savings).
2. Barriers and problems (decreased student interaction, technological shortcomings).

Table 1. Summary of Research Reviewed

Author	Title	Type of Distance Education	Sample	Purpose	Findings
Armstrong, Toebe and Watson (1985)	Strengthening the instructional role in self-directed learning activities	Print: Correspondence	RNs	To determine what factors contribute to learner participation and completion of self-directed study courses in continuing nursing education.	Incorporation of many of the personal/social aspects of traditional learning by specific instructional strategies and enhancement of the course facilitator role did provide effective interaction with course materials, thus leading to successful self-directed course completion.
Bernard and Naidu (1990)	Enhancing interpersonal communication in distance education: Can "voice-mail" help?	Audio: Voice-mail telephone-based communication system	Nondegree RNs	To determine need for voice-mail support for print-based distance education courses.	The results suggest that communication is occurring between and among students in the program; respondents' reaction to the potential usefulness of the proposal system of voice-mail communication in the program was extremely favorable.
Billings (1987)[a]	Factors related to progress toward completion of correspondence courses in a baccalaureate nursing program.	Print: correspondence course	BSN	To develop a model of completion of correspondence courses that identifies factors related to progress toward course completion.	Students most likely to make progress towards course completion in 3 months submit the first lesson within 40 days of receiving the course materials, have a high SAT and GPA, have completed other correspondence courses (and not dropped courses), receive family support, and probably is not working, and does not require the support of employer.

Billings (1992)	Computer conferencing: The role of the nurse in health education in a distance learning environment	Computer conference	High school students, nursing faculty	To determine the effectiveness of the computer conference as a model for health education and to identify the role of the nurse.	Descriptive study showed that types of communications, categories, and themes of questions indicate students have varied needs for health information. The role of the nurse in an "electronic school district" is expanded, and central to health instruction.
Boyd and Baker (1987)	Using television to teach	Television; Teleconferencing	MSN students	To assess academic achievement of students enrolled in TV courses, compared with on-campus courses.	In this evaluation, students in TV courses had higher GPA's; more students in TV courses graduated than on campus.
Chick & Paull (1988)	Collaboration between nurse educators in Australia and New Zealand extends educational opportunities for nurses	Print: learning package	Post RNs-BSN Students	To evaluate effectiveness of a collaborative endeavor between nurse educators in New Zealand and Australia combining their resources for the benefit of students and faculty in both settings.	Case study showed that cooperative course endeavors speeds development. Course development between faculty at 2 schools in different countries is possible; lack of faculty release time produces frustration.
Colbert (1984)	Nursing management in the 80's: A seven-part teleconference series	Television: Teleconference	RNs	To determine if teleconferencing is a viable means to educate and inform health care professionals.	Results of the evaluation questionnaire showed teleconferencing as a viable means to deliver instructional information to health care professionals.

Table 1. (*Continued*)

Author	Title	Type of Distance Education	Sample	Purpose	Findings
Cragg (1991)	Professional resocialization of post-RN baccalaureate students by distance education	Mixed: audio teleconference/print (correspondence)	Post RN Baccalaureate Students	To determine if professional resocialization is effective using a distance education approach.	Distance courses can be influential in the professional resocialization of post-RN students.
Fulmer, Hazzard, Jones, & Keene (1992)	Distance learning: An innovative approach to nursing education	Television: Teleconference	RNs non-degree	To determine views of nursing departments' experience with distance learning technologies.	Off-campus students achieved higher course grades than on-campus students.
Goldrick, Appling, Stevens, & Larson (1990)[b]	Infection control programmed instruction: An alternative to classroom instruction in baccalaureate nursing education	Print: Self-managed learning-form of programmed unit of Instruction (PUI)	Baccalaureate Nursing Students (3rd yr)	To determine whether self-managed learning in the form of a programmed unit of instruction is an acceptable alternative for teaching infection control to nursing students.	This experimental study indicated that nursing students who complete an infection control PUI score higher on post-tests than those who attend a lecture (P.001) regardless of pretest scores and educational setting.
Guillemin (1984)	Assessment of learning needs and interest in distance education technology of southern rural Alberta nondegreed registered nurses	Television: Teleconferencing	Nondegree RNs	To assess the learning needs of nondegree RNs with respect to interest in credit courses for a Bachelor of Nursing degree and the utility of delivering	This survey indicated that nurses in rural Alberta are interested in credit courses for a BSN degree through teleconferencing.

				these credit courses through a distance delivery system of teleconferencing.	
Huckaby (1981)[c]	The effects of modularized instruction and traditional teaching techniques on cognitive learning and affective behaviors of student nurses	Print: modularized instruction	Student nurses	To meet the increasing educational needs of students with diverse abilities and speeds of learning.	Modular group learned significantly more than the lecture group. Modular/lecture group demonstrated significantly more affective behavior than the modular alone group. The lecture group demonstrated significantly more affective behaviors than the modular group.
Keck (1992)	Comparison of learning outcomes between graduate students in telecourses and those in traditional classrooms	Television: Teleconference	MSN Students	To compare learning outcomes between students taught by TV and those taking the classes in a traditional classroom.	Students at remote sites achieved course grades comparable to those in the studio who had closer contact with the professor in the TV studio.
Kuramoto (1984)	Teleconferencing for nurses: Evaluating its effectiveness	Mixed: audio/print/on-site faculty	RNs	To develop and compare alternative methods for delivering continuing nursing education.	A statewide distribution system using three methods of course delivery is effective in terms of increasing participants' cognitive knowledge, as well as nurses' learning and satisfaction.
Luchsinger (1990)	Distance education in the mountain plains states for associate degree nursing programs	Mixed: Television; videotaped instruction; Audio-graphic teleconferencing Audio tele-	ADN Students	To determine the utilization of distance education by Associate Degree Nursing programs in the mountain plains states.	There were no differences in outcomes; in some cases those students off campus achieved higher scores.

Table 1. (*Continued*)

Author	Title	Type of Distance Education	Sample	Purpose	Findings
		conferencing; cable networking computer managed instruction/ conferencing			
McClelland and Daly (1991)	A comparison of selected demographic characteristics and academic performance of on-campus and satellite-center RNs: Implications for the curriculum	Mixed: Satellite Center using audiotapes, videotapes, and correspondence study	RN-BSN students	To compare and contrast certain demographic characteristics of RN students enrolled on campus with those enrolled in outreach satellite centers.	Demographic profile differences revealed that the RN students in satellite centers were slightly older, were employed, worked more hours per week; they tended to work full-time, traveled further to attend classes, had more children and took longer to complete the BSN course. Satellite center RN students had higher ACT-PEP mean scores and transfer GPA's than their on-campus peers. The students in the satellite areas received lower grades.
Moser & Kondracki (1977)	Comparison of attitudes and cognitive achievement of nursing students in three instructional strategies	Television: television vs lecture method	Freshman nursing students	To compare the attitudes and the cognitive achievement of nursing students exposed to three instructional strategies.	There was a preference for and greater interest in color video tapes than in black and white TV. A comparison of TV vs traditional lecture method in terms of cognitive achievement failed to yield significant differences.

Nikolajski (1992)	Investigating the effectiveness of self-learning packages in staff development	Print: self learning packages	RNs	To determine if the use of self-learning packages is an alternative to traditional in-service programs.	Nurses using the self-learning package had a mean knowledge increase of 19.5% as opposed to a 34% knowledge increase among nurses who attended traditional in-service programs.
Parkinson & Parkinson (1989)	A comparative study between interactive television and traditional lecture course offerings for nursing students	Television: Videoconference	LPNs pursing ADN	To determine if differences existed between ITV students in the following three areas: 1) perception of instructor's effectiveness, 2) perception of course content, and 3) examination scores.	Results indicated the live teacher was preferred. There were no significant differences in the examination scores. ITV group rated the material content and course difficulty as significantly "overloaded" and too challenging.
Phillips, Hagenbuch, & Baldwin (1992)	A collaborative effort in using telecommunications to enhance learning	Television: teleconference	RNs, LPNs Nursing Assistant's other medical personnel	To determine the instructional needs of RNs, LPNs and other personnel involved in patient care.	Survey findings identified teleconferencing as an acceptable vehicle for providing courses for certification review and continuing education for RNs and for providing courses for college credit leading to a variety of degrees in nursing.
Rufo (1985)	Effectiveness of self-instructional packages in staff development activities	Print: self-instructional packages (SLP)	RNs	To determine if learning gained from self-instruction and from lectures and/or demonstration were equal	5 out of 10 SLPs proved to be significantly effective. 3 out of 10 SLP indicated with some changes and re-evaluation can be significantly effective. Remaining 2 SLP showed there was less learning in the self-instructional format.
Russell (1990)[d]	Relationships among preferences for	Mixed: Print/ Audiotape/	RNs	To determine relationships of preference for	As need for structure increases, self-directed readiness decreases;

Table 1. (*Continued*)

Author	Title	Type of Distance Education	Sample	Purpose	Findings
	educational structure, self-directed learning, instructional methods, and achievement	Modules vs lecture		structure, self-directed learning use of modules vs lecture, and achievement.	neither need for structure or self-directed readiness predict achievement. There were no differences in achievement for students preferring low structure when using the modules or attending lecture.
Sanborn, Sanborn, Seibert, Welsh, & Pyke (1973)	Continuing education for nurses via interactive closed-circuit television: A pilot study	Television: Teleconference	RNs	To determine the acceptance of two-way, closed-circuit TV as a medium of continuing education for RNs	Questionnaire results indicate a relatively strong acceptance of the medium by nurses as a means of continuing education
Scheele, Smith, & Perry (1992)	Telecommunications and in-service training of nurse managers: Evaluating a distance model	Television: teleconference	Nurse managers	To determine preference for different training topics as well as preferred delivery systems.	The data from the questionnaire reveal that utilizing teleconferencing for training for first and second level nurse supervisors was preferred but the most preferred topics do not lend themselves to teleconferencing.
Thiele & Higgs (1992)	Distance learning: Developing and conducting thesis research via computerized communication network	Computer: Computer conferencing	RNs pursuing a Master's Degree	To determine if students are able to pursue graduate study from a distant site.	Faculty were able to successfully guide the development of a thesis via a computer.

Thompson & Taylor (1991)	"Well, was it worth it?" The value of teletutorials for bachelor of nursing students	Audio: Audioconference telephone tutorials	RNs pursuing BSN	To evaluate teletutorial support for correspondence courses.	Teletutorials provided a sense of belonging to a group and a forum for discussion.
Viverais-Dresler & Kutschke (1992)	RN students' satisfaction with clinical teaching in a distance education program	Television: teleconference	RN/BSN mobility program	To investigate student satisfaction of clinical courses by distance education.	Satisfaction with the clinical teacher's role was high; both quantitative and qualitative data indicate respondents felt a positive and supportive relationship with the clinical teacher.
Wiley (1983)	Effects of a self-directed learning project and preference for structure on self-directed learning readiness	Print: modules	BSN Students	To examine the effects of preference for structure and a self-directed learning project on the SDL readiness of junior-baccalaureate nursing students.	Because of trait-treatment interaction, teaching the SDL process to all nursing students does not result in an overall increase in these students' ability to direct their own learning; those who prefer low structure benefit from SDL teaching, but those who prefer high structure do not benefit from the type of SDL teaching utilized in this study.

Theoretical framework is relevant for the sources noted:
[a] Bean's synthetic model of student attrition from institutions of higher education.
[b] Reinforcement theory.
[c] Motivation and locus of control.
[d] Mocker and Spear's concept of control.

3. Outcomes (academic achievement, satisfaction, socialization and affective outcomes, participation and attendance, course and degree completion).
4. Clinical instruction.
5. Learner support (experience, readiness, learning style).
6. Faculty role and workload.

Advantages and Benefits of Distance Education

Authors of articles on distance education tend to be favorable toward this form of education. Both supporting and research-based articles cite access to education, recruitment and retention, and cost savings as the primary advantages of distance education.

Access. One of the greatest benefits of distance education is access to both basic and continuing nursing education by students who are geographically dispersed (DeSilets, 1986; Wieseke & Pavlechko, (1992). Access also refers to convenience and flexibility, which are particularly important as nurses return to school while they continue with their work and family responsibilities (Lowis & Ellington, 1991). For students at a distance, having access to courses and faculty decreases a sense of isolation (Thompson & Taylor, 1991). Secondary benefits may be anonymity and decreased fear of risk in participating in class (Billings, 1992).

For a variety of reasons, access to distance education courses and programs is appealing to nurses and nursing students. Nursing students tend to be older, employed, carrying family responsibilities, and living at great distances from campuses offering nursing degree programs (McClelland & Daly, 1991; Osborne & Dow, 1989). Registered nurses use distance education courses to improve professional knowledge and skills (Armstrong, Toebe, & Watson, 1985; Clark, 1986; Rufo, 1985) as well as for professional advancement—relicensure, college credit toward degrees, certification programs, and continuing nursing education.

Recruitment and retention. Distance education is a mechanism for recruitment (Billings, Frazier, Lausch, & McCarty, 1989; Boyd & Baker, 1987; Collins, 1987) and retention for schools of nursing and nursing service. When students can take courses at hospitals, they have opportunities to increase their qualifications for employment (Maltby, Drew, & Andrusyszyn, 1991) and, because they can continue to work, there is decreased turnover (Collins, 1987). Because students can study at their own pace, they can also continue to be employed (Haggard, 1992).

Cost savings. Cost savings is also cited as an advantage of using distance education. Although costs are reported in various ways, distance education courses can be cost-effective, and participants are often willing to support the costs (Colbert, 1984).

In print-based instruction, development costs (teacher time, typing, duplicating, and so on) are offset by savings in teaching time and materials (Nikolajski, 1992). Rufo (1985) concluded that there is decreased instructor burnout because instructor expertise is used, and increased job satisfaction because instructors can be creative. Cost savings also accrue when learning time is decreased, as in the case of programmed instruction (Goldrick et al., 1990). Distance education saves travel time and expense for faculty and students. DuGas and Casey (1987) estimated that offering courses by distance education costs one-third less than sending faculty to teach in two remote sites.

Television-based instruction, on the other hand, is costly when on-air time, faculty development and faculty teaching expense, development and distribution of supporting materials, mailing, reception site management, equipment and studio time are considered (Clark & Cleveland, 1984; Fulmer, Hazzard, Jones, & Keene, 1992). These up-front costs can be offset by using statewide broadcast systems or consortial arrangements. Phillips et al. (1992) reported that costs for continuing education courses break even when production costs can be offset by large enrollments at reception sites. Fulmer et al. (1992) reported cost savings using microwave (one-way video) transmission rather than two-way television when broadcasting credit courses in a BSN program.

Maximizing faculty time and expertise is also cost-effective when there is a shortage of faculty and large numbers of students need access to well-prepared faculty (Fulmer et al. 1992; Nikolajski, 1992).

Barriers and Problems

Distance education, despite its many advantages, also has drawbacks. Two problems consistently noted in the literature are: (1) decreased student interaction and (2) technological shortcomings (of a variety of media).

Decreased student interaction. Faculty and students value the classroom exchanges that occur in traditional classroom settings. These are typically lost or need to be supported in other ways, when courses are offered as distance education. For example, Cragg (1991) noted limits of interaction in print media because, with correspondence instruction, dialogue occurs only between student and faculty and there is no opportunity for peer interaction and socialization.

Technological shortcomings. The electronic technologies supporting distance education are not perfect (Sanborn, Sanborn, Seibert, Welsh, & Pyke, 1973). For example, there is frustration on the part of the students and faculty when the video and audio components of the television transmission system break down (Boyd & Baker, 1987; DuGas & Casy, 1987; Phillips et al., 1992).

Outcomes

The research indicates that academic outcomes of distance education are generally positive. Course achievement and satisfaction with instruction reach levels comparable to those in traditional classrooms. Where technological and distance barriers to learner support and socialization exist, faculty use a variety of compensating strategies.

Academic achievement. The primary purpose of most studies of distance education in nursing has been to determine academic achievement and ensure comparable learning outcomes for courses/lessons/modules. Comparing videoteleconferencing with lecture in an introductory pathophysiology course for LPNs, Parkinson and Parkinson (1989) found no significant differences in course grades. Moser and Kondracki (1977) also found no significant differences in cognitive achievement between BSN students taking a televised course and BSN students in traditional lecture courses. Using a telephone interview to ascertain exam results for ADN students at three reception sites in an eight-state area, Luchsinger (1990) found no difference in course grades between those students taking the course via television and those on-campus. Keck (1992) also found no significant differences between course grades for MSN students who were in a traditional on-campus statistics course and those who received the course by closed-circuit television around the state; furthermore, there were no differences in final course grades between students who took the class in the television studio and students who attended reception sites.

McClelland and Daly (1991), reporting on student achievement differences between on-campus and distance education found that students at the distance campus had higher GPAs than students on campus, but the students did not receive higher grades in the Foundations of Nursing Practice course. However, these findings were attributed to the fact that off-campus students were employed more, drove farther to class, and had more family responsibilities than the students taking the on-campus course. Fulmer et al. (1992) also found that BSN students taking a class by teleconference had higher grades than students on campus.

Similar positive learning outcomes are reported for print-based instruction. Russell (1990) found no difference in achievement on posttest scores for students using a module or attending a lecture on the same content. Goldrick et al. (1990) found that students using a programmed instruction module scored higher than students receiving the content by lecture. Nikolajski (1992), on the other hand, found that knowledge gain was less when nurses used self-learning packages as opposed to a traditional in-service program, and attributed this finding to lack of familiarity with self-learning methods or lack of match with learning style.

Huckaby (1981), using an experimental design, compared differences of module, lecture plus module, and lecture alone with MSN students in a nursing education course. Groups were matched for GPA, age, and marital status, and were studied over three different semesters. Students in all three instructional delivery systems learned; there were no significant differences between students in the module and module-plus-lecture groups, but students in the module groups did learn more than those in the lecture group. Huckaby (1981) concluded that the independent study module is adequate to achieve course objectives. Rufo (1985) found that the experimental group using self-instructional packages had posttest scores that were higher for most modules, but the extent of gain varied by unit and topic when compared with lecture alone.

Comparable learning outcomes have been obtained in audio-based courses. Comparing posttest results of nurses enrolled in five continuing education courses offered with a teacher in the classroom, with a teacher in a two-way audio class, or as independent study, Kuramoto (1984) found no significant differences in cognitive knowledge. Additionally, of the three methods, the audioconference contributed to 40 percent of the registration in the five courses.

Satisfaction. Researchers also investigated student satisfaction with the experience of distance education. Most studies are designed to compare satisfaction with distance education with response to traditional on-site education. Results are mixed.

For print-based systems, Goldrick et al. (1990) investigated BSN student satisfaction with a programmed unit of instruction (PUI); students did not find using the PUI more complex than attending a lecture, and, in fact, preferred this format. In Huckaby's (1981) study, students preferred the module plus lecture more than the lecture or module alone; they valued the direct contact with faculty.

Students also tend to be satisfied with the medium of television for receiving noncredit courses. Moser and Kondracki (1977) found learner satisfaction with television was not less than with on-campus lecture, but students did prefer color television to black-and-white.

Two studies investigated satisfaction with faculty in distance education. Fulmer et al. (1992) reported that having multiple teachers presenting the telecourse frustrates students. Parkinson and Parkinson (1989) indicated that students were less favorable toward the television instructor and preferred the live teacher.

Kuramoto (1984), comparing independent study, audioconferencing, and an on-site teacher, found that there were significant differences in attitude toward the delivery system, but differences occurred on a course-by-course basis. When students in a continuing education course received via cable television responded to an evaluation questionnaire, 90 percent liked viewing the course by television (Clark & Cleveland, 1984). Colbert (1984), in evaluating a teleconference series for health care administrators, found that 73 percent of the participants found television to be a good delivery method for content in their field.

Socialization and affective outcomes. Socialization into the profession and the development of professional values are important components of nursing education. Although faculty use a variety of teaching strategies to promote these affective outcomes, the research suggests that socialization is easier with television and audio-based delivery systems than it is with print-based delivery systems.

Cragg (1991), in a telephone interview with 24 students, investigated the extent of socialization of RN-BSN students enrolled in a nursing issues course at four universities. Two of the courses were delivered by audioconference and two were offered by correspondence. In this study, there were no significant differences in socialization to the profession. Any differences were attributed to the instructor and the attitude of the institution toward its distance students. Boyd and Baker (1987) reported that, according to informal evidence in a MSN program offered by teleconference, student socialization occurs when students form study groups, faculty invite students to campus for discussion groups, and students become members of the graduate student organization.

Strategies to ensure socialization can be designed in lesson-courses. Thompson and Taylor (1991) increased student–faculty interaction with teletutorial support for a course offered by audioconference. Cragg (1991) also reported that the peer group is important in socialization to the profession; students in an audioconference course had more peer support than students in correspondence courses.

Participation and attendance. Learning occurs when students are actively involved. Factors that contribute to attendance and participation in distance education include access to and availability of instruction and instructional technology that supports student–faculty and peer interaction. Fulmer et al. (1992) noted that students are initially uncomfortable in participating in class discussion in television courses, and they need orientation and encouragement from faculty. Nikolajski (1992) found that, when in-service programs were offered by self-learning packages rather than by traditional unit in-service programs, staff nurses participated more; evening and night shifts participated more in the self-learning method than did the day shift. Kuramoto (1984) studied differences in registration as an indication of participation in continuing education courses offered by independent study, audioconference, and with an on-site teacher. There was greater registration in the independent study method (53 percent) and audioconference (40 percent) than in the on-site lecture (15 percent). There was also increased attendance at the course delivered by audioconferencing, which indicates that the physical presence of the teacher is not necessary to ensure attendance.

Student participation in distance education classes can be facilitated by faculty. Students participate more when given an orientation session on how to study or participate using the medium (Fulmer et al., 1992; Lowis & Ellington, 1991; Wuest, 1989). Wuest (1989) found that, in a class offered by audioconference, one student tended to speak for the group; she recommended that faculty solicit contribution from individuals as well as groups. Wuest (1989), comparing students in the studio classroom with those at reception sites, found that there was increased participation by students in the studio, leading to frustration on the part of students at the reception site. Faculty can encourage individual student participation in TV courses by calling on students specifically (DuGas & Casey, 1987; Fulmer et al., 1992; Wuest, 1989; Wurzbach, 1993). Interactive teaching–learning strategies such as discussion, debate, and ice-breaker exercises also help engage students in the class (Wuest, 1989). Other strategies include using photographs of students at reception sites to personalize participation (Wurzbach, 1993). Pym (1992), commenting from a feminist perspective on class participation, reported that women students find contact with the teacher important; the support within and between groups of students is also helpful.

The classroom environment facilitates participation. When using audio-based technologies, the room must be quiet (Thompson & Taylor, 1991). The teacher must take care that the environment is not disruptive. Thompson and Taylor (1991) found that a class size of about seven students is ideal for participation; smaller groups place undue demands for participation on students and faculty. Furthermore, students need convenient access to microphones at the reception sites, in order to participate easily (Fulmer et al., 1992; Wuest, 1989).

Course and degree completion. Although the primary advantage of distance education is to increase access for geographically distant learners, this benefit is lost if students do not complete courses and degree programs. A variety of factors influences progress toward completion, but the findings related to success are mixed.

Dropout has been a major problem with print-based distance education. Billings (1987) investigated progress toward course completion for BSN students in correspondence courses and found that completion of the courses was related to high SAT and GPA and to when students started the courses. Students tended to complete the courses if they started within three months of enrolling in the course; other significant factors were family support, previous experience with correspondence courses, and goals for degree completion.

Armstrong et al. (1985) used self-directed modules to provide seven continuing education courses to nurses in Alaska. Course completion ranged from 28 percent to 100 percent. Course completion was enhanced by a facilitator who provided lesson feedback and telephone contact; the completion rate improved when learners started the course within two weeks of receiving course materials, and declined when work and family pressures increased.

Kuramoto (1984) found attrition rates varied among delivery methods as well as among courses; course attrition increased with the self-study delivery method and was attributed to the motivation required to complete the course. Huckaby (1981), in a study of 32 MSN students, found that one-sixth of students enrolled in a module-only version of the courses dropped out. Students in this study indicated that they missed contact with the faculty. In this same study, students preferred the module-plus-lecture. Thus, although students preferred the self-paced features of the module, they also preferred a relationship with a faculty.

For their MSN television courses, Boyd and Baker (1987) reported that graduation rates are higher for students in telecourses and progress toward completion is faster than for students on campus. McClelland and Daly (1991), on the other hand, found that the BSN students on a satellite campus using mixed-media delivery systems projected a longer time to complete the BSN degree program than did those on campus. This can be attributed to the demographic differences of the students on the satellite campus, who tend to be older, working, and carrying family responsibilities. Clark and Cleveland (1984) reported that, of the 86 nurses enrolled in a six-hour cable telecourse for continuing education credit, only 64 percent of those registered completed the course and received the certificate.

Clinical Instruction

Although most research focuses on the effects of didactic instruction, nursing is an applied, practice-based profession. Because clinical experiences are difficult to arrange at a distance, offering entire degree programs is difficult. The challenge is to find clinical facilities near the student and employ prepared clinical instruction/preceptors who are well-oriented to their responsibilities and committed to the program. Faculty from the college or university offering the course or program are responsible for the final evaluation, which may be conducted in collaboration with the on-site adjunct faculty or preceptor.

There are several models for offering clinical instruction at a distance. One approach is to employ on-site clinical faculty. In an

RN-BSN program (Viverais-Dresler & Kutschke, 1992), the university hires on-site clinical faculty. The faculty from the university orient the clinical faculty and provide ongoing support through telephone conferences. Gallagher (1984) reported the benefits of supporting on-site clinical faculty through teleconferences. Student satisfaction with clinical faculty was high, but unfamiliarity with the clinical setting and role changes caused difficulty for the students (Viverais-Dresler & Kutschke, 1992). Clinical faculty also have been employed as adjunct faculty for an RN-BSN course offered by independent study (Lethbridge, 1988). Students keep clinical logs and submit them to the campus faculty; students use their own hospitals and must meet the same clinical objectives, but they do not need to invest the same amount of time in clinical practice.

In another model, faculty from the campus travel to the distance education clinical sites (Major & Shane, 1991). Faculty may modify clinical supervision, but they maintain the same number of contact hours as in the on-campus course. Differences in clinical course outcomes are not reported for either model.

Learner Support

For many students, learning at a distance involves a change from expectations in traditional classroom settings. Faculty must assess learner readiness for distance education, prepare students to use technology, and match learning styles with the demands of the delivery system.

Experience/Readiness. Distance education requires students to be independent and self-sufficient in order to overcome technological and separation barriers. Most research suggests students need orientation to distance education regardless of the technology. For example, it is important to orient students to television and the studio prior to their experience in the studio and at the reception site (Billings et al., 1989; Clarke & Cohen, 1992).

Wuest (1989) found that students who were experienced with audioconferencing were able to help orient newcomers. Hamilton and Gregor (1986) used a learning contract to help registered nurses use a self-directed learning program. Billings (1987) found that students who had taken previous correspondence courses were more likely to make progress toward completion of subsequent courses. However, Russell (1990) found that there was no difference in self-directed readiness, preference, and achievement when BSN students used a learning module compared to a lecture.

Advisement and recruitment are important adjuncts to distance education systems. Thiele and Higgs (1992) reported the frustration of students who were connected to faculty only by computer conference.

Learning style. Teaching and learning involve complex interactions among the learner, the setting, and the instruction. These relationships are critical when traditional instruction is modified for students at a distance (Billings, 1991). For example, structure, the preference for guidance or explicit directions about how to study, is often absent or limited with distance education. Wiley (1983) investigated the effects of a self-directed learning project and preference for structure on self-directed learning readiness. In this study, two experimental groups conducted an independent learning project and two control groups followed traditional teacher-directed learning. Preference for structure was measured using Ginther's Reaction to Statements (RTS), and self-directed readiness was measured using Guglielmino's Self-Directed Learning Readiness Scale (SDLRS). Wiley (1983) found that neither preference for structure nor self-directed learning readiness contributed to variance, but interaction of the two variables accounted for modest variance, and students who prefer low structure benefit from SDL more than those who prefer high structure. Russell (1990) also used the RTS and SDLRS to identify differences in readiness and structure for students using a learning module compared with students attending a lecture. Russell (1990) found that, as the need for structure increased, self-directed learning readiness decreased, but neither was able to predict achievement in the learning unit.

Faculty Role and Workload

Although not a primary focus of the research-based articles, the role of faculty is described in several supporting articles as "changing." Teaching at a distance requires adaptation of course materials, additional preparation time, and modification of teaching and evaluation strategies. Faculty must adapt teaching style for the medium (Billings et al., 1986; Billings et al., 1989; Boyd & Baker, 1987). For example, faculty teaching on television must be friendlier and more supportive, to overcome barriers (Parkinson & Parkinson, 1989).

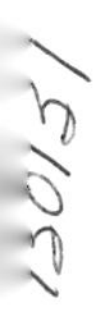

Faculty workload is also identified as an issue. Boyd and Baker (1987) provided released time for course preparation during the semester before teaching a television class. When there is no workload adjustment, faculty are frustrated, but they can maximize workload if they team-teach and collaborate in development of materials (Chick & Paull, 1988).

The faculty role is changing from provider of instruction to instructional designer (Billings, 1992; Billings et al., 1986; Lowis & Ellington, 1991); conference moderator (Billings, 1992; Thiele & Higgs, 1992); and facilitator (Thompson & Taylor, 1991). Support for role changes and impact on an academic career are not, however, reported in the nursing literature.

SUMMARY

An increasing body of research literature reveals that technological advances in distance education delivery systems provide opportunities for increasing access to nursing education, maximizing limited instructional resources, sharing faculty expertise, and overcoming barriers of distance and time. This review has identified how faculty in schools of nursing and staff development educators in a variety of health care agencies are utilizing distance education to provide instruction. In spite of the limitations of the research, several conclusions and recommendations for additional research about distance education can be drawn from this review.

CONCLUSIONS

The review of research indicates that, regardless of the delivery system, learning outcomes are generally equivalent when distance education is compared with traditional classroom instruction. Academic achievement, as measured by lesson and course grades, has not been shown to be different and in some instances may be improved. Other learning outcomes such as learner satisfaction and socialization are also positive. However, program/course/lesson completion is more of a problem (1) for print-based technologies and (2) when the learners are not enrolled in courses/lessons with fixed time limits (semesters) or teacher-directed courses.

The costs of distance education are not well understood or clearly reported, but distance education appears to be cost-effective when resources are contributed or shared and when large enrollments support course development. The front-end costs of print-based technologies are less than video-based or audio-based delivery systems and can often be more easily justified.

Learners in distance education programs require considerable support. Students must be oriented to the medium and encouraged to participate in class discussion, particularly in television-based courses. Faculty can use a variety of strategies to provide "high-touch" activities that will ensure socialization and other affective outcomes. For example, faculty can require students to come to the campus or studio classroom for one class session, hold on-campus course orientations prior to the start of class, and/or have an end-of-course party during which students and faculty can meet each other. Other strategies include having "office hours" on-line immediately following the televised class, using toll-free numbers to ensure easy student access to faculty.

The teaching role of faculty is changing. Although only a few studies investigated the changed teaching activities or perceptions of faculty teaching using distance education technologies, it is clear that faculty must adapt teaching and evaluation strategies to the distance delivery medium. For example, when teaching on television, faculty must modify discussion strategies to accommodate students at a distance and develop visual aids that use large print. When designing print-based courses, faculty must structure learning experiences that can be accomplished outside of the traditional classroom. Thus, there is increased workload as courses are developed or adapted for distance education.

This review did not reveal discussions of political and policy implications such as, who "owns" the class presentation, especially when videotaped by those who "receive" the class at a remote site. As administrators, faculty, and students become dependent on distance education technologies for course delivery, issues of access to resources, ethics of use, and policy development will likely surface. These issues are being raised in other arenas and are important to nurse educators as well.

RECOMMENDATIONS FOR FURTHER RESEARCH

As nurse educators advance the agenda for nursing and nursing education reform, teaching and learning at a distance will be one way to ensure educational access and effective use of limited instructional resources in restructured educational environments. Building on the previous research, which has answered questions about learning outcomes and satisfaction, additional questions can be raised to further understanding about the role and effectiveness of distance education in nursing education. A sampling of these questions follows:

1. *The faculty.* Little is known about the experience of teaching in distance education. How is the teaching role changed? What faculty development is necessary to support faculty? Who are the innovative teachers and how can they be supported and rewarded? How can student–faculty relationships be nurtured? What encourages mentoring at a distance? How is faculty scholarship demonstrated in distance education teaching?
2. *Students.* Student roles change in distance education, and learner support is needed to orient students and encourage class/course participation. Additional information is needed about peer support and collaborative learning. What is the effect of a learner-centered system of education? Who are the learners? Do they reflect the diversity of communities served by the educational institution? What additional needs do learners have?
3. *Outcomes.* Given the current emphasis on educational outcomes, research in distance education can continue to answer questions about course and program outcomes. However, since questions about cognitive outcomes have been answered, additional research should focus on acquisition of information-processing skills such as critical thinking, clinical decision making, collaboration, cooperation, and conflict resolution. What is the impact of distance education on the development of these skills? What teaching strategies used in distance education courses effectively develop these skills? Outcomes of students' retention and graduation can also be investigated in terms of the impact of various delivery systems. For example, does the contact with faculty and structure provided by televised courses improve the poor course completion rates noted for print-based delivery systems?
4. *Delivery systems.* Additional understanding is needed about the appropriate mix of delivery systems for specific learners and content. Answers are needed to questions about models of distance education and clinical instruction. As education reforms focus on the community as practice setting, can distance education contribute to basic education and nursing staff development in these clinical practice settings? Can distance

education in community-based settings more closely align practice and education?

5. *Methodological concerns.* Future research must attend to methodological deficits noted earlier. Researchers should describe carefully the setting and the delivery system; delivery systems and teaching strategies must be clearly differentiated. Case studies and other qualitative designs can contribute to eliciting answers to questions arising from the experience of distance education for students, faculty, and administrators. Finally, the research should be theoretically grounded.

REFERENCES

Armstrong, M. L., Toebe, D. M., & Watson M. R. (1985). Strengthening the instructional role in self-directed learning activities. *The Journal of Continuing Education in Nursing, 16*(3), 75–84.

Arndt, M. J. (1990). Nursing education via the airwaves. *Nurse Educator, 15*(1), 10.

Bailey, C., (1987a). Nursing distance education in Alberta: a preliminary history, Part 1. *Alberta Association of Registered Nurses Newsletter, 43*(1), 13–15.

Bailey C., (1987b). Nursing distance education in Alberta: a preliminary history, Part 2. *Alberta Association of Registered Nurses Newsletter, 43*(2), 15–17.

Bernard, R. M., & Naidu, S. (1990). Enhancing interpersonal communication in distance education: Can "voice-mail" help? *Educational and Training Technology International, 27*(3), 293–300.

Billings, D. M. (1987). Factors related to progress toward completion of correspondence courses in a baccalaureate nursing program. *Journal of Advanced Nursing, 12,* 743–750.

Billings, D. (1991). *Student learning style preferences and distance education: A review of literature and implications for future research.* The Second Symposium on Research in Distance Education, The Pennsylvania State University, May 22–24.

Billings, D. (1992). Computer conferencing: The role of the nurse in health education in a distance learning environment. In N. Estes & M. Thomas (Eds.), *The Ninth International Conference on Technology and Education, Paris, France, Vol. 3* (pp. 1393–1395). Austin: The University of Texas at Austin, College of Education.

Billings, D., Frazier, H., Lausch, J., & McCarty, J. (1989). Videoteleconferencing: Solving mobility and recruitment problems. *Nurse Educator, 14*(2), 12–16.

Billings, D. M., Marriner, A., & Smith, L. (1986). Correspondence courses: An alternative instructional method. *Nurse Educator, 11*(4), 31–37.

Boyd, S., & Baker, C. M. (1987). Using television to teach. *Nursing and Health Care, 8*(9), 523–527.

Brunt, B., & Scott, A. L. (1986). Factors to consider in the development of self-instructional materials. *The Journal of Continuing Education in Nursing, 17*(3), 87–93.

Carey, R. L. (1988). Athabasca University: Distance education in nursing. *Alberta Association of Registered Nurses Newsletter, 44*(8), 19–20.

Chick, N., & Paull, D. (1988). Collaboration between nurse educators in Australia and New Zealand extends educational opportunities for nurses. *International Journal of Nursing Studies, 25*(4), 279–286.

Clark, C. E. (1989, May/June). Telecourses for nursing staff development. *Journal of Nursing Staff Development,* 107–110.

Clark, C. E., & Cleveland, T. L. (1984). The media and the mode. *The Journal of Continuing Education in Nursing, 15*(5), 168–172.

Clark, K. M. (1986). Recent developments in self-directed learning. *The Journal of Continuing Education in Nursing, 17*(3), 76–80.

Clarke, L. M., & Cohen, J. A. (1992). Distance learning: New partnerships for nursing in rural areas. *Rural Health Nursing,* 359–388.

Colbert, C. D. (1984). Nursing management in the 80's: A seven-part teleconference series. In L. A. Parker & C. H. Olgren (Eds.), *Teleconferencing and Electronic Communications III.* Madison, WI: Center for Interactive Programs, University of Wisconsin Extension.

Collins, F. (1987). Reaching out. *RNABC News, 19*(5), 24–26.

Cragg, C. E. (1991). Professional resocialization of post-RN baccalaureate students by distance education. *Journal of Nursing Education, 30*(6), 256–260.

DeJonge, J., & McDougall, L. (1989). Inter-university collaboration in the development of a distance education course in community health nursing. *Journal of Nursing Education, 28*(7), 325–327.

DeSilets, L. (1986). Self-directed learning in voluntary and mandatory continuing education programs. *The Journal of Continuing Education in Nursing, 17*(3), 81–83.

Dow, M. E. (1988). Distance education for nursing at the University of Calgary. *Alberta Association of Registered Nurses Newsletter, 44*(8), 10.

DuGas, B. W., & Casey, A. M. (1987). Teleconferencing. *The Canadian Nurse,* 22–25.

Dyck, S., (1986). Self-directed learning for the RN in a baccalaureate program. *The Journal of Continuing Education in Nursing, 17*(6), 194–197.

Fulmer, J., Hazzard M., Jones, S., & Keene, K. (1992). Distance learning: An innovative approach to nursing education. *Journal of Professional Nursing, 8*(5), 289–294.

Goldrick, B., Appling-Stevens, S., & Larson, E. (1990). Infection control programmed instruction: An alternative to classroom instruction in baccalaureate nursing education. *Journal of Nursing Education, 29*(1), 20–25.

Guillemin, E. (1984). Assessment of learning needs and interest in distance education technology of southern rural Alberta nondegreed registered nurses. *Alberta Association of Registered Nurses Newsletter, 40*(5), 25–26.

Guillemin, E. J. (1986). Outreach post-R.N. degree program: A demonstration project. *Alberta Association of Registered Nurses, 42*(1), 6–8.

Haggard, A. (1992). Using self-studies to meet JCAHO requirements. *Journal of Nursing Staff Development, 8*(4), 170–173.

Hamilton, L., & Gregor, F. (1986). Self-directed learning in a critical care nursing program. *The Journal of Continuing Education in Nursing, 17*(3), 94–99.

Hast, A. S. (1987). Self-learning packages in critical care. *Critical Care Nurse, 7*(2), 110–116.

Heath, J. (1991). Open learning in health care settings. *Nursing Standard, 5*(35), 37–39.

Henry, P. (1993). Distance learning through audioconferencing, *Nurse Educator, 18*(2), 23–26.

Huckaby, L. (1981). The effects of modularized instruction and traditional teaching techniques on cognitive learning and affective behaviors of student nurses. *Advances in Nursing Science, 33,* 67–82.

Keck, J. F. (1992). Comparison of learning outcomes between graduate students in telecourses and those in traditional classrooms. *Journal of Nursing Education, 31*(5), 229–234.

Kerr, J. C. (1987). History of off-campus programs and distance education at the University of Alberta. *Alberta Association of Registered Nurses Newsletter, 43*(93), 19–20.

Kerr, J. R. (1988). Nursing education at a distance: Using technology to advantage in undergraduate and graduate degree programs in Alberta, Canada. *International Journal of Nursing Studies, 25*(4), 301–306.

Kleinknecht, M. K., & Hefferin, E. A. (1990). Maximizing nursing staff development—the learning laboratory. *Journal of Nursing Staff Development,* September/October, 219–224.

Kuramoto, A. (1984). Teleconferencing for nurses: Evaluating its effectiveness. In L. A. Parker & C. H. Olgren (Eds.), *Teleconferencing and Electronic Communications III.* 262–268. Madison, WI: Center for Interactive Programs, University of Wisconsin Extension.

Lethbridge, D. (1988). Independent study: A strategy for providing baccalaureate education for RNs in rural settings. *Journal of Nursing Education, 27*(4), 183–185.

Limón, S., Spencer, J. B., & Henderson, F. C. (1985, June). Video-teleconferencing by nurses—for nurses. *Nursing & Health Care,* 313–317.

Lowis, A., & Ellington, H. (1991). Innovations in occupational health nursing education, including a distance learning approach. *American Association of Occupational Health Nursing Journal, 39*(7), 316–318.

Luchsinger, B. (1990). Distance education in the mountain plains states for associate degree nursing programs. *Journal of Adult Education, 19*(1), 13–18.

Major, M. B., & Shane, D. L. (1991). Use of interactive television for outreach nursing education. *The American Journal of Distance Education, 5*(1), 57–66.

Maltby, H., Drew, L., & Andrusyszyn, M. A. (1991). Distance education: Joining forces to meet the challenge. *The Journal of Continuing Education in Nursing, 22*(3), 119–122.

McClelland, E., & Daly, J. (1991). A comparison of selected demographic characteristics and academic performance of on-campus and satellite-center RNs: Implications for the curriculum. *Journal of Nursing Education, 30*(6), 261–266.

Moser, D. H., & Kondracki, M. R. (1977). Comparison of attitudes and cognitive achievement of nursing students in three instructional strategies. *Journal of Nursing Education, 16*(1), 14–28.

Muse, C. T. (1984). Teleconferencing continuing medical education, continuing nursing education, and other health related programs. In L. A. Parker & C. H. Olgren (Eds.), *Teleconferencing and Electronic Communications III.* Madison, WI: Center for Interactive Programs, University of Wisconsin Extension.

Nikolajski, P. Y. (1992). Investigating the effectiveness of self-learning packages in staff development. *Journal of Nursing Staff Development, 8*(4), 179–183.

Osborne, M., & Dow, M. (1989). The mature learner and distance education. *Alberta Association of Registered Nurses Newsletter, 45*(4), 15–16.

Parkinson, C. F., & Parkinson, S. B. (1989). A comparative study between interactive television and traditional lecture course offerings for nursing students. *Nursing & Health Care, 10*(9), 499–502.

Phillips, C. Y., Hagenbuch, E. G., & Baldwin, P. J. (1992). A collaborative effort in using telecommunications to enhance learning. *The Journal of Continuing Education in Nursing, 23*(3), 134–138.

Pym, F. R. (1992). Women and distance education: a nursing perspective. *Journal of Advanced Nursing, 17,* 383–389.

Reilly, D. E. (1990). *Graduate professional education through outreach: A nursing case study.* New York: National League for Nursing.

Roe, S. C. (1991). Decentralizing education facilitates academic pursuits for nurses. *Aspen's Advisor for Nurse Executives, 7*(1), 6–8.

Rufo, K. L. (1985). Effectiveness of self-instructional packages in staff development activities. *Journal of Continuing Education in Nursing, 16*(3), 80–83.

Russell, J. M. (1990). Relationships among preferences for educational structure, self-directed learning, instructional methods, and achievement. *Journal of Professional Nursing, 6*(2), 86–93.

Sanborn, D. E., Sanborn, C. J., Siebert, D. J., Welsh, G. W., & Pyke, H. F. (1973). Continuing education for nurses via interactive closed-circuit television: A pilot study. *Nursing Research, 22*(5), 448–451.

Scheele, R., Smith, J. B., & Perry, R. T. (1992). Telecommunications and in-service training of nurse managers: Evaluating a distance model. In N. Estes & M. Thomas (Eds.), *The Ninth International Conference on Technology and Education, Paris, France, Vol. 3* (pp. 90–92). Austin: The University of Texas at Austin, College of Education.

Thiele, J. E., & Higgs, Z. R. (1992). Distance learning: Developing and conducting thesis research via computerized communication network (case study). In N. Estes & M. Thomas (Eds.), *The Ninth International Conference on Technology and Education, Paris, France, Vol. 3* (pp. 1329–1330). Austin: The University of Texas at Austin, College of Education.

Thompson, D., & Taylor, B. (1991). "Well, was it worth it?" The value of teletutorials for bachelor of nursing students. *The Australian Journal of Advanced Nursing, 8*(2), 27–33.

Tribulski, J. A., & Frank, C. (1987, Summer). Closed circuit TV: An alternate teaching strategy. *Journal of Nursing Staff Development,* 110–115.

Viverais-Dresler, G., & Kutschke, M. (1992). RN students' satisfaction with clinical teaching in a distance education program. *The Journal of Continuing Education in Nursing, 23*(5), 224–230.

Wieseke, A., & Pavlechko, G. (1992). A model for open and distance learning for RN baccalaureate nursing students (videocase study). In N. Estes & M. Thomas (Eds.), *The Ninth International Conference on Technology and Education, Paris, France, Vol. 3* (pp. 1063–1065). Austin: The University of Texas at Austin, College of Education.

Wiley, K. (1983). Effects of a self-directed learning project and preference for structure on self-directed learning readiness. *Nursing Research, 32*(3), 181–185.

Wuest, J. (1989). Debate: A strategy for increasing interaction in audio teleconferencing. *Journal of Advanced Nursing 14,* 847–852.

Wurzbach, M. E. (1993). Teaching nursing ethics on interactive television: Fostering interactivity. *Journal of Nursing Education. 32*(1), 37–39.

Chapter Two

CARING: CURRICULAR ISSUES

Betsy Frank, RN, PhD

INTRODUCTION

In 1986, advocates of curriculum revolution in nursing education declared their efforts as having begun (Tanner, 1990b). This revolution was predicated on the need to transform nursing curricula to better meet the demands of the changing health care environment. Often called the Caring Curriculum Movement, it was spawned by the Society for Research in Nursing Education (now the Council for Research in Nursing Education within the National League for Nursing). The Fourth Annual National League for Nursing's Conference on Nursing Education gave credence to this movement. The conference, held in 1987, was entitled, "Curriculum Revolution: Mandate for Change." At that conference, Bevis (1988) stated that nursing programs based on behavioristic models were merely technical training programs, not professional education programs. She also stated that a professional education should nurture the caring role. In 1989, Bevis further explicated her ideas in a book co-authored with noted educator Jean Watson, *Toward a Caring Curriculum: A New Pedagogy for Nursing*. Moccia, an original advocate for the curriculum revolution, has also elucidated the major elements of the Caring Curriculum. At the 1987 conference, Moccia (1988) called for nursing educators and nurses in the service arena to reclaim the caring tradition that once was a part of nursing's heritage, but was and is in danger of being lost in the current society, which values high technology. Tanner (1990a) also supported Bevis's contention that caring is a core value of the curriculum revolution movement.

Since 1987, several other League-sponsored conferences have addressed the concerns of this curricular movement, providing a forum for sharing research findings from studies that have dealt with these concerns. Now, seven years later, it is time to analyze and synthesize findings from the studies presented at these conferences, as well as other published research. If, indeed, caring underpins nursing's epistemology (Watson, 1990), and if caring truly is a proper value orientation in teaching (Noddings, 1988), then a status report

Table 1. Studies Reviewed for Caring: Curricular Issues

Author/Date	Data Collection Method	Data Analysis Method	Sample
Students and Faculty: Perceptions of Caring			
Diekelmann, 1989	Interviews	Hermeneutical inquiry	Generic BSN and RN BS students (number not reported)
Eriksson, 1989	Questionnaire	*t*-test	63 Swedish graduate students
Nelms, 1990	Semistructured interview	Phenomenological	17 BSN students
Chipman, 1991	Written critical incidents, follow-up interviews	Constant comparative	26 second-year diploma students
Mangold, 1991	Care Q questionnaire	Man–Whitney U	30 senior BSN students, 30 RNs
Kelly, 1991	Interviews	Constant comparative	12 British fourth-year undergraduates
Kelly, 1992a	Interviews	Constant comparative	23 senior BSN students
Kelly, 1992b	Interviews	Constant comparative	23 senior BSN students
Komorita, Doehring & Hirchert, 1991	Care Q questionnaire	Kruskal–Wallis	113 master's-prepared educators, managers, clinical specialists
Student–Faculty Interactions			
Stephenson, 1984	Semistructured Interview	Grounded theory	22 British students, 23 nurse tutors (2 schools)
Berman, 1988	Interviews, observation	Ethnographic and interpretive	Second-semester ADN clinical group
Miller, Haber, & Byrne, 1990	Open-ended interviews	Phenomenological	6 senior BSN students, 6 faculty
Appleton, 1990	Open-ended interviews	Phenomenological	2 doctoral students
Halldorsdottir, 1990	Open-ended interviews	Phenomenological/ Grounded theory	9 former Icelandic BSN students

Beck, 1991	Written descriptions	Phenomenological	4 junior and senior BSN students
Students' Perceptions of Uncaring Behaviors			
Hughes, 1992	Semistructured interview	General qualitative	10 BSN students (5 schools)
Theis, 1986	Unstructured questionnaire	Categorized data according to a priori categories	204 BSN students (3 schools)
Pagana, 1988	Open-ended questionnaire (20 items) Threat scale	ANOVA descriptive statistics, general discussion of written comments	262 BSN students (7 schools)
Caring Content within Nursing Curricula			
Slevin & Harper, 1987	Open-ended and forced-choice questionnaire	Content analysis, descriptive statistics	273 BSN programs
Bauer, 1990	Open-ended interviews Examination of documents		26 faculty, 32 BSN students (5 schools)
Evaluation of Caring as a Learning Outcome			
LaMonica, 1983	Empathy training program	Not described	Not described
Rogers, 1986	Empathy Construct Rating Scale (ECRS)	ANOVA, factor analysis	135 junior and senior BSN students (2 programs), 135 patients
Norris, 1986	Quasi-experimental	ANOVA, ANCOVA	147 sophomore BSN students
Forsyth, Delaney, Maloney, Kubesh, & Story, 1989	Formative and summative evaluation techniques	Not described	124 nursing alumni and employers, BSN students at all levels

of our current understanding of caring within educational environments is essential for further development of current curricular trends.

To accomplish this critical review of the caring curriculum research, a MEDLINE search using the terms "caring—teaching and modeling within the college of nursing" was carried out. Kuhn (1970) suggested that a shift in thinking may be evident in a discipline's writings before an actual paradigm change occurs. With this in mind, the MEDLINE search began with the year 1983. Pertinent references mentioned in the articles located through the MEDLINE search, but not listed in that search, were also retrieved. Not surprisingly, most of the studies have been published since 1986. However, a few studies, reported before the revolution's declaration, focused on constructs such as empathy, which could be construed as a part of caring.

Articles retrieved were placed into two categories: (1) student–faculty interactions and (2) curricular issues. Uncertainties and gaps in the research were identified, and future research directions were suggested. Table 1 lists the articles reviewed.

STUDENT–FACULTY INTERACTIONS

Some nursing educators are moving away from a behavioristic educational model. Inherent in this move is a belief that students are unique beings who are respected and valued (Tanner, 1990b). Nursing education, then, becomes an interpersonal shared process between student and teacher (Sheston, 1990). Students often choose nursing because they want to care for others (Kersten, Bakewell, & Meyer, 1991). As de Tornay (1990) has argued, student–faculty partnerships can help model this sense of caring that students expect. Therefore, analyzing the nature of student–teacher interactions is essential.

Students and Faculty: Perceptions of Caring

Diekelmann (1989) used hermeneutical inquiry to describe the lived experiences of nursing students. Her particular report summarizes findings from several studies. One theme that came from her studies was "learning as evaluation." She noted the adversarial nature of evaluation. Anger and frustration were evident in the extensive narrative accounts provided. Diekelmann stated that perhaps these data showed current teaching practices seek to change technical and intellectual skills rather than to transform one's understanding of what it means to care for patients.

Another of Diekelmann's studies (reported in this same article) confirmed and extended her work. Registered nurses (RNs) returning to school equated learning with evaluation. Additionally, RN students had difficulty seeing how their practice experiences had transformed their understanding of causal relationships. Data from RN students also revealed a theme of "being in practice and returning to school." These students faced incredible pressures to cope with the demands of their personal, professional, and student lives.

In conclusion, Diekelmann stated that, by using hermeneutical inquiry, students and teachers can engage in dialogue. As a result, they may be open to many possibilities that will facilitate, in a phenomenological sense, the understanding required to learn about and give nursing care. She went on to say that this understanding would help to transform the curriculum from a behavioristic to a more caring approach.

Eriksson's (1989) report of her research demonstrated that students across different cultures could identify caring concerns. She investigated what paradigm students began their education with, how the paradigm changed during their education, and what paradigm was evident upon completion of the curriculum. Data were collected via a questionnaire based on Torneboehm's caring paradigm. Five competencies were a part of this framework: (1) cultural, (2) linguistic, (3) communicative, (4) social (acknowledging respect for others), and (5) sociocultural. Sixty-three graduate students at the Swedish School of Nursing in Helsinki comprised the study's sample. The five-point Likert-scale questionnaire was administered at the beginning and at the end of the program. No description of the questionnaire's reliability or validity was given. Twelve questions from the competence profile were listed; whether these constituted the total questionnaire was uncertain. Further, the questions were not identified for which of the five competencies they belonged to.

Forty-nine students identified the link between caring practice and caring science; nine students thought the relationship was unclear, and five had not experienced any such relationship. Caring competencies were measured for all 63 students when they began their program, but only 34 students had competencies measured at the end. No reason was given for the dropouts. The author stated, however, that the beginning caring competencies of the 34 who completed the study were no different from the total group who began the study. Further, once data were analyzed regarding competencies upon initial enrollment in the program, curriculum was changed to strengthen linguistic and communicative competencies. At the beginning of the program, students identified their ability to perform specialized nursing activities as very good. Sociocultural competencies were also rated as good, but communicative and linguistic capabilities were rated only satisfactory or fair. Upon graduation, changes in students' competencies were significant ($p < 0.001$) for all factors except giving specialized care ($p < .05$). Communicative and linguistic competencies improved the most. This finding was to be expected, especially given the fact that the curriculum was changed between the two data collection points specifically to enhance these particular skills.

Nelms (1990) interviewed 17 students at a southern university who were at various points in their BSN nursing curriculum. The eight interview questions posed were described in the research report. From the data collected, Nelms sought to "provide a theoretical base on which nursing education could incorporate the lived experience of nursing students into its curriculum through phenomenological methodology" (p. 286). No particular phenomenological methodology was cited. And, given that Nelms stated she had used a phenomenological approach, some researchers may question her use of the extensive semistructured interview technique.

Nelms concluded that being a student was a life-pervasive commitment. Students saw clinical experiences in general and caring as the core of nursing; they expected faculty to be caring, competent, and supportive, and to recognize them as human beings. Fellow students provided the most support and caring. Faculty, nursing staff, families, and friends outside of nursing provided support as well, but students felt their lived experiences were not understood by these groups. Short quotes were given to support these conclusions.

Chipman (1991) asked 26 second-year diploma students for written descriptions of critical incidents involving nursing behaviors that could have been described as caring or noncaring. Follow-up interviews were conducted to clarify and amplify written material. Her overall purpose was to help determine what caring content needed to be included in a proposed new curriculum based on Jean Watson's theoretical framework. Data were analyzed using a constant comparative method, although no particular methodology was cited. Findings showed that students thought caring was giving of self, meeting patients' needs in a timely manner, and providing for comfort. The author demonstrated the themes through the use of illustrative quotes. Noncaring behaviors were described as the opposites of the caring behaviors identified above. Chipman concluded that students could describe caring as more than technical competence. Thus, the author stated that the curriculum should include humanistic as well as technical knowledge.

Mangold's (1991) study demonstrated that students and practicing nurses have similar beliefs about the importance of caring behaviors. Thirty senior baccalaureate students from one school and 30 professional nurses with more than one year of experience (educational preparation not identified) completed the 50-item, 6-subscale CARE-Q instrument. The subscales were: (1) accessible, (2) explains and facilitates, (3) comforts, (4) anticipates, (5) trusting relationship, and (6) monitors and follows through. Face and content validity of this instrument have been established. Test–retest reliability in previous studies was 79.1 percent for the most important caring behavior and 63.4 percent for the least important caring behavior. No reliability statistics were mentioned for Mangold's study sample. The Mann Whitney U was used for data analysis. Results showed that the students and practicing nurses showed no difference in the overall rankings of importance of identified caring behaviors, with the exception of the trusting behaviors. Nurses rated trusting behaviors slightly higher, but the difference only approached statistical significance ($p < .06$). The author noted that this difference may have been due to the fact that the trust subscale of the CARE-Q had more items than the other five subscales and, thus, was more discriminating. The author also pointed out that the older average age of the professional nurses (six years' difference) may have impacted this finding.

Both students and nurses agreed that "listening to the patient" was the most important caring behavior. Students thought the least important behaviors (ranked equally) were "puts patient first, no matter what," "is professional in appearance," "volunteers to do little things," and "suggests questions to the doctors." The practicing nurses identified "professional appearance" as the least important behavior. One could conclude that the low ranking of "doing the little things" contradicted Chipman's findings. However, this appeared not to be the case. Students in Mangold's study did rank the comfort measures subscale (nine items) the highest. Comfort could include "doing the little things." Of concern is that both students and practicing nurses ranked professional appearance the lowest. Indeed, Mangum, Garrison, Lind, Thackery, and Wyatt (1991) have reported that patients do value nurses' appearance.

One could question the parochial nature of Mangum et al.'s sample. Nevertheless, the importance of professional appearance warrants further exploration.

Kelly (1991) studied British fourth-year undergraduate nursing students. Twelve students from two institutions served as informants. Initial questions from the audiotaped interviews focused on the definition of professional values. Although no theoretical structure was derived, data were analyzed using the constant comparative methodology from Glaser and Strauss's (1973) grounded theory approach. Kelly demonstrated that standards were equated with values, and the two standards most identified were "respect" and "taking time for little things." Both standards have been identified as parts of the larger construct of caring (Chipman, 1991). One should note, however, that Kelly (1990) separated respect from caring. Themes that emerged supported the notion that caring is a cross-cultural concern. Further, the data from the British study (Kelly, 1991) showed that students were concerned that their values might not be in step with the real world. The data presented herein verified this contention.

Kelly (1992a, 1992b) also reported on two separate aspects of data collected from what appears to be one study. Twenty-three seniors from a class of 120 students in the final clinical rotation of a BSN program were the study's subjects. Data reported in the first article (1992a) were collected through audiotaped semistructured interviews and clinical diaries. The author again stated that analysis occurred using the constant comparative methodology from Glaser and Strauss's (1973) grounded theory approach; however, no theoretical structure was derived from these data either. Informants were given the opportunity to validate the findings following preliminary data analysis. In addition, two experts were used to verify the conclusions reached from the raw data. The data in response to the question, "What do you believe good nursing is . . . ?" (Kelly, 1992a, p. 12) showed that respect and caring were central to good nursing. Illustrative quotes were quite helpful in elucidating these central themes. The author, however, concluded that the students were out of step with the realities of actual practice. One wonders how the author came to that conclusion; unlike Kelly (1991), supportive data were not presented. One could also question whether this conclusion actually biased the data analysis that led to this opinion.

From the same data set, Kelly (1992b) explored the perceptions of self-concept and the influential sources for the development of self-concept. Only audiotaped interviews were used for the data collection for this portion of Kelly's study. As with the other data, the constant comparative methodology from the grounded theory approach was used to analyze the data. Participant and expert validation of findings occurred. Again, no theoretical structure was derived.

Informants identified themselves as caring, but lacked confidence in their technical skills. Some students did, however, see themselves as both caring and competent. One might speculate whether students, in this study, did not see competence as a part of caring. Good role models, who were primarily nursing faculty and clinicians (although some did mention family and friends), were those who were supportive and took time to listen. The author pointed out that students did describe themselves in terms similar to their role models. She was unsure whether the students came to the program with many of the identified qualities of a good nurse or whether they emulated their role models. She noted that nursing faculty seemed to have a very powerful influence on their students. As with the other reported findings, illustrative quotes supported the identified themes gleaned from the data.

Faculty Perceptions of Caring

One study specifically addressed faculty members', as well as other master's-prepared nurses' perceptions of caring. Komorita, Doehring and Hirchert (1991) used the CARE-Q to identify faculty perceptions of caring behaviors and to compare their perceptions to other master's-prepared nurses. The same test–retest reliability statistics cited by Mangold were used for this instrument. All but three (110 of 113) nurses with master's degrees who lived in a particular region of a midwestern state answered the questionnaire. Seventy-two educators, 13 managers, and 23 clinical specialists participated in the study. Because there was no difference in rankings of most important behaviors between educators and nurses in the other functional areas, the authors stated the data were combined for analytical purposes. The Kruskal–Wallis statistic was used to compare the least important behavior item rankings between various groups such as educators versus other nurses and medical-surgical educators versus other educators. Specific items that ranked the highest across all groups included "is calm," "checks out with patient the best time to talk with the patient about his/her condition," and "gives patient's treatments and medications on time." Group differences were noted when least important behaviors were analyzed. For example, educators thought "is cheerful" ($p < .05$) was less important than did other groups. Using data published elsewhere, the researchers also compared their findings to patients' perceptions of caring. Although no statistical significance could be computed, of particular note was the fact that patients ranked technical behaviors higher than did the respondents in Komorita et al.'s study (1991). Similar to the students and patients in Mangold's (1991) study, these participants highly ranked comfort measures.

Student–Faculty Interactions

Identification of caring behaviors by students and faculty facilitates the understanding of the concept of caring in general. Knowing how the caring behaviors occur within the educational arena *between* faculty and students can help faculty and students have a vision of how the curriculum might be better transformed from a behavioral to a more caring model.

Stephenson (1984), in a pre-curriculum revolution study, investigated the student–nurse tutor (instructor) relationship. Twenty-two British nursing students and 23 nurse tutors from two hospital schools of nursing participated in the study. Data were collected using a semistructured interview format and were analyzed through a grounded theory approach. The questionnaire framework was not described. However, role theory may have formed the basis for the questions used, because role theory was discussed in the background of the study.

Students said that tutors should be friendly, but not too friendly. Students also commented that being overly friendly could cause the tutor to lose group control, and that tutors had too little time to build a relationship with students.

Mutual trust and respect were rated as important by both students and faculty. Tutors and students alike stressed the need for tutors to act in a caring manner toward students. However, tutors identified organizational constraints, such as the need to consult with supervisors or to record in students' records the nature of the students' personal and academic problems. Tutors said they sometimes ignored these organizational requirements.

One strength of this study was the fact that Stephenson (1984) did propose a theoretical framework grounded in the collected data. She suggested that the ideal student–tutor relationship was built on mutual trust and respect, on a proper amount of friendliness, which allows the tutor to counsel or discipline students as needed, and on the competence of the tutor.

Berman (1988), a professor of education administration, conducted a most unique study. Her purpose was to lend an outsider's perspective to the teaching of caring. She collected 60 hours' data using ethnographic and interpretive techniques. Initially, Berman sought to evaluate evidence of caring in students and faculty. She also wanted to discover what meaning these behaviors had for the students and the instructor who were observed. One instructor and a group of second-semester associate degree students were the subjects for this exploration. As the study progressed, the investigator began to move away from the original study questions to consider the dilemmas that faced the students and the instructor. Such a change in focus is not uncommon in studies that use ethnographic and interpretive methods. Because data collection and analysis occur simultaneously, the researcher can change direction if the data warrant.

The novice students had fragile self-images. To them, caring meant being with patients or having face-to-face contact, but not doing care plans. Students felt that they should feel comfortable in caring with all types of patients, but felt less than adequate with some groups of patients, such as the elderly. Students often had to reconcile what was learned in class with the dynamics of the real world. Because students were enrolled in an integrated curriculum, they felt frustrated by the need to adjust on a daily basis to new clinical settings.

The instructor was faced with dilemmas of her own. She had to negotiate between patients' and students' needs. The instructor recognized that time limitations often hampered the students' ability to establish caring relationships with patients.

Berman concluded that dilemmas were an inherent part of teaching caring within the clinical environment. She proposed that these dilemmas presented opportunities for creative teaching and learning.

In a more recent study, Miller, Haber, and Byrne (1990) also explored caring within student–teacher interactions from both student and faculty perspectives. Six senior nursing students and six faculty who had taught for more than three years were study participants. Open-ended interviews were conducted by three different researchers. Subjects were randomly assigned to the interviewers.

The question that began the interviews was reported. Phenomenological methods suggested by Giorgi (1985) and Colaizzi (1978), as well as others, guided the data analysis. One unique facet of this study was that the three researchers analyzed all the interview data individually. Then they met to synthesize their results and to write the phenomenological descriptions. Study participants were given an opportunity to validate the written descriptions. Of note is the authors' statement that, after interviews with three faculty and three students, caring themes emerged. However, the planned six additional interviews were conducted to ensure that premature study closure did not occur.

Students summarized caring interactions by saying they took place within an entire climate of support. Faculty had a holistic concern for students and reached out to students in an empathetic manner. Students and faculty had mutual trust and connectedness.

Faculty, on the other hand, characterized caring as an interactive process that took place within a caring philosophical framework. For faculty, caring was the essence of the student–faculty relationship. Faculty also placed caring within a holistic framework.

Three other investigators (Appleton, 1990; Beck, 1991; Halldorsdottir, 1990) also studied perceptions of faculty–student interactions from a phenomenological perspective. These researchers, however, explored only the students' perception of the caring encounters.

Appleton (1990) utilized a phenomenological approach characterized by Ray (1987) to describe two doctoral students' perceptions of the meaning of caring within the academic setting. Interviews, portrayed as open dialogues, generated the data. The author said that she assessed the study's credibility using the criteria outlined by Lincoln and Guba (1985); yet she did not provide specific evidence of her study's credibility.

A table, within the article that reported the research findings, clearly outlined the derived themes. Supportive quotations explicated the caring process the students experienced. The themes shown were commitment, involvement, and belonging. The data demonstrated that students developed relationships with faculty and other students that facilitated personal and professional growth. An example of an expression of caring was "being treated with respect."

The second study involved subjects from a country outside the United States. Halldorsdottir (1990) investigated the essential structure of a caring student–faculty encounter by interviewing nine former Icelandic BSN students. The author stated that a phenomenological approach was used to guide the choice of the study sample and to direct the unstructured interview process. The researcher stressed that the subjects were co-researchers and, through dialogue, the critical nature of caring as well as uncaring student–teacher encounters was described. However, the investigator further said that a constant comparative method was used for data analysis. Methodological purists might question this approach (Morse, 1991). Unlike Stephenson's and others' approaches, Halldorsdottir interviewed only former, not current students (with the exception of one doctoral student). Similar themes could be found within all these studies.

The former BSN students stated that professional competence, genuine concern for the student as a scholar, a positive personality, and a professional commitment were part of a caring student–teacher relationship. Mutual trust was also important, and six stages of a working relationship were described. Like the students in other studies, particularly Stephenson's (1984), these participants stressed the need for students and teachers to have a respectful distance between personal and professional relationships. For these former students, a caring interaction resulted in a sense of self-worth, personal and professional growth, appreciation and role modeling, and long-term caring and respect. Uncaring was characterized as lack of professional competence, lack of concern, demand for control, and destructive behavior. Following the conventions of grounded theory, Halldorsdottir placed the findings within a theoretical framework that depicted the essential nature of a caring student–faculty interaction. Extensive sample quotes were not provided to substantiate the identified themes.

Beck (1991) used written descriptions from 47 junior and senior BSN nursing students to construct a picture of caring student–teacher interactions. Students were asked to recount an incident in which they had felt a faculty member was caring. The respondents were asked to describe thoughts, perceptions, and feelings. Using Colaizzi's (1978) methodology, themes were identified. Significant statements depicted the themes of attentive presence, sharing of self, and consequences. The author concluded that the themes gave credence to Roach's (1984) five C's of caring: (1) compassion, (2) commitment, (3) competence, (4) confidence, and (5) conscience.

One final study also delineated the students' perspective on student–faculty interactions within a caring climate. Hughes (1992) used audiotaped interviews to examine these interactions.

She began each interview by asking students to describe the atmosphere in their school. Nine other questions guided the interview's structure. The junior nursing students (two each from five different schools) served as the study's informants. Data were analyzed by placing statements into categories and subcategories. The procedures used for category identification were not stated. The author further said that, two weeks following the original data analysis, a random sample of 20 percent of cards on which data statements were recorded was reanalyzed by the investigator and two nurse educators. Cohen's Kappa for intrarater reliability was 96; for interrater reliability, K = .83. As data were analyzed, the researcher came to the conclusion that the categories from her study were similar to themes identified by Noddings (1988). Study participants identified a climate of caring as one in which modeling, dialogue, practice of caring behaviors, and confirmation took place. Data examples substantiated the identified themes. This particular study was unusual in the fact that the author seemed to be extending a previously developed theoretical framework through qualitative methods. Additionally, the author collected data from more than one school. However, the author did not describe the use of any particular framework for analysis other than a general qualitative methodology.

Students' Perceptions of Uncaring Behaviors

Student respondents in several of the aforementioned studies (for example, Halldorsdottir, 1990) did identify uncaring behaviors experienced in encounters with faculty, but two studies focused exclusively on these uncaring behaviors. Theis (1986) gathered data from 204 senior nursing students from three different baccalaureate programs. The number asked to participate in the study was not mentioned, but the author reported that three blank questionnaires were returned. In an unstructured questionnaire, the students were asked to describe teaching behaviors they considered unethical. Data were classified according to a priori categories of respect for persons, justice, and beneficence.

Educators would like to think that the majority, if not all, of their encounters with students are ethical; however, only 17 percent of study respondents reported *no* unethical encounters. Fourteen percent of the unethical encounters involved non-nursing faculty. Quotations from the students' written responses unfortunately supported the fact that some faculty lacked respect for students, were unfair, and did cause harm to students and perhaps to patients. All of these behaviors could be construed as uncaring as well as unethical, in that ethical comportment is a part of caring (Kelly, 1990).

Pagana (1988) used the cognitive appraisal of stress theory as a basis for having students identify threats and challenges within the clinical teaching environment. The data collection instrument consisted of open-ended questions (number unidentified), followed by a 20-item scale to measure threat and challenges. The psychometric properties were reported in the author's dissertation and, thus, were unavailable to the average reader. Drawn from seven different BSN programs, 262 students who were in their first medical-surgical nursing course participated in the study. Whether this number comprised the total sample available was not reported.

Results showed students were more challenged than stressed. Of particular interest to this discussion of uncaring student–faculty encounters, however, was the fact that the content analysis of the qualitative data demonstrated that 26 percent of the students viewed the clinical instructor as a threat. Two particular colleges accounted for the majority of these comments. Students questioned their instructors' competence, were threatened by the constant questioning, and perceived the instructor as impatient. The author concluded that the information from this study might sensitize faculty to the fact that students do encounter threats, which, as Diekelmann (1989) pointed out, are a part of the lived experiences of students. However, Pagana (1988) suggested that faculty could perhaps mediate part of the stress encountered through positive interactions with students.

CURRICULUM ISSUES: CONTENT AND OUTCOMES

Understanding how faculty and students define and perceive caring within educational settings is important. Just as important is knowing what is being taught in regard to caring and describing the learning outcomes. Acquisition of this knowledge can assist both faculty and students to design curricula that are less behavioristic and concomitantly more caring in nature.

Caring Content within Nursing Curricula

Slevin and Harper (1987) surveyed 273 of 450 accredited baccalaureate and higher-degree nursing programs. The content of the survey focused on whether caring was taught, how it was taught, and how it was evaluated, and on whether faculty caring skills were addressed. Sixty-one percent responded to open-ended and forced-choice questions. Of particular interest is the fact that these data were collected prior to the official beginning of the caring curriculum movement. One should note, then, that survey respondents may have defined caring in a different manner from educators and others who have, since 1986, been exposed to literature that specifically emphasizes caring within educational environments. Over 97 percent of the surveyed schools included caring content in their curricula, and over 70 percent integrated the content throughout. Twenty-six percent singled out the concept of caring for discussion.

The authors assumed the presence of this caring content through the answers to questions dealing with constructs such as stress, empathy, and trust. Content related to caring was found primarily in the junior and senior years. This finding was to be expected, given the fact that the majority of nursing courses are taught in the junior and senior years of BSN programs. Content was presented in lectures and assigned readings, and through process recordings. Evaluation occurred by using tests, case studies, and care plans. One hundred fifty-eight schools reported experiences used to facilitate the faculty's promotion of caring. Student evaluation tools were employed by more than 80 percent of the schools to evaluate faculty caring behaviors.

More recently, Bauer (1990) studied, in depth, how caring was addressed in baccalaureate curricula. Open-ended interview data were collected from 26 faculty and 32 senior students at five schools where caring was a central focus in the curricula. In addition, curricular documents were examined. The author stated that a phenomenological approach was used to guide the study, but no particular methodology was elucidated.

Working from the assumption that a philosophy guides a curriculum's framework, the philosophies from the five schools were examined. Caring was viewed as an interpersonal process and as the essence of nursing. End-program objectives, course content, and learning strategies reflected this belief. Content themes identified included: caring about self and others, holistic care, attributes of caring, skills emphasizing caring, nursing process, and discussion of research focused on caring. Faculty behaviors facilitated the teaching of caring. Identified behaviors included: instilling feelings of self-worth in students, being available, and role modeling. Selected anticipated outcomes were nurses' feeling more satisfied, patients' expressing positive responses, and students' internalizing the value of caring. Informants cautioned, however, that caring could be physically and emotionally exhausting.

Evaluation of Caring as a Learning Outcome

Evaluating learning outcomes is difficult. Most research examines evidence of learning within the short term. LaMonica (1983) outlined in detail a 16-hour empathy-training course. Empathy, as defined by LaMonica, includes caring attitudes and behaviors such as sensitivity and being present in relationships with others. The rationale given for the course was that empathy is central to a helping relationship. Although no research design was reported, LaMonica stated that preliminary research results supported the effectiveness of this program.

Three investigators jointly presented evidence that specific caring communication skills could be taught. Friedrich, Lively, and Schacht (1985) used the Egan communication model to teach communication skills to students enrolled in an integrated curriculum. Forty students enrolled in a psychiatric nursing course participated in a 12-hour training program. Prior to undertaking this course, faculty assessed audiotapes of students' interactions with patients. Faculty concluded that, based on Carkhuff's (1969) scale, students had minimal empathic responses. Following the skills training, students' audiotapes showed a growth in empathic responses.

Rogers (1986) built on LaMonica's work when she measured students' empathy ratings. Empathy was examined in sophomore, junior, and senior BSN students from two different programs. Two hundred five students completed the 84-item LaMonica Empathy Construct Rating Scale (ECRS). However, only 135 questionnaires were used because the other respondents had had previous nursing education at the LPN or ADN levels. Additionally, 135 patients cared for by the students were asked to complete the ECRS. Cronbach's alpha reported from LaMonica's work was $r = .96$ for self-report and $r = .97$ for client ratings. Factor analysis from Rogers' study showed two factors. They were named (1) compassion and (2) insensitivity/indifference.

Students had moderately well-developed empathy ratings. The mean for the self-report was 175.4. Patients rated students slightly higher: 188.7. Possible scores for the ECRS ranged from -252 (absence of empathy) to $+252$. The correlation between the students' self-report rating and the patients' rating of the students was significant at the $p < .001$ level. When one compares these findings with those of Friedrich et al. (1985), one might wonder if the students in Friedrich's study were all that different from those in Rogers' study. However, Rogers used a questionnaire to collect data, and Friedrich et al. used actual audiotaped interactions to evaluate empathic responses. Thus, differences in empathy ratings reported by Friedrich et al. may have been due to the evaluation methods used.

Rogers (1986) also reported that student empathy ratings in one school increased throughout their program, although the increase was statistically nonsignificant. In the other school, the ratings decreased somewhat. Rogers suggested that a cultural effect may have come into play. In that school, the junior class contained a large minority urban population and an influx of Haitian immigrants. Students' day-to-day living conditions may have influenced their empathy ratings. One might conclude from these findings that students come to schools of nursing with an empathic nature, and the curriculum has the potential for reinforcing this value.

Norris (1986) compared two methods for teaching communication skills. One hundred forty-seven sophomore students were randomly assigned to a lecture or role-playing group for the purposes of learning communication skills. Both groups shared common readings and videotapes. Based on Carkhuff (1969), concepts within the course for both groups included respect, caring, concreteness, and empathy. Results indicated that males learned more through role play ($p < .05$) than through lecture. The investigators stated that gender differences could be attributed to sex-role socialization. However, this finding may have been spurious because the authors intimated that the numbers of males involved were small. Students in the role-playing group were more involved in their learning. Students who were field-independent learners performed better on the objective tests, no matter which group they were in. From this study, one might conclude that faculty should attempt to use a variety of strategies to teach caring content, thereby accommodating different learning styles.

Forsyth, Delaney, Maloney, Kubesh, and Story (1989) assessed more global learning outcomes. Using formative and summative evaluation techniques, they demonstrated that caring could indeed be taught. An example of a specific evaluation tool was given in this rather general summary report of findings from several research studies. Of particular interest was the fact that employers rated the majority of graduates' caring behaviors "excellent" or "above average" on a four-point Likert scale. This scale included measures of clinical expertise (presumably defined as technical expertise). Although the research account gave minimal detail regarding the research designs, it gave credence to the notion that evidence of caring could be evaluated.

DISCUSSION

The curriculum revolution has certainly engendered much research concerned with caring in educational environments. Studies published prior to 1986, as well as studies reported during the first two or three years of the revolution, indicated that a curriculum paradigm shift was occurring prior to the revolution's declaration.

A variety of methodologies have been used to study the elusive concept of caring. Some investigators who chose to study a component of caring, such as empathy, used quantitative methodologies to answer their research questions. Caring in a more global sense was also studied using quantitative methods. Established instruments were used; however, the researchers did not give reliability statistics for the samples used in their studies. They relied, instead, on previously reported reliability statistics.

Phenomenological, ethnographic, constant comparative, and grounded theory approaches were also used to explore caring issues. Some authors, such as Hughes (1992), used a more nondescript qualitative approach to data gathering and analysis; others, such as Berman (1988), combined several methods to gather and collect data. Expert qualitative researchers would probably find fault with both Hughes's and Berman's methodological choices.

Studies that presented extensive quotations to substantiate conclusions were most useful. As Diekelmann (1991) has suggested, the narrative truly is a powerful tool for understanding the realities of students and faculty within nursing programs. Moreover, when the methodology was more fully described, the reader could better judge the study's rigor; the study conducted by Miller et al. (1990) was such a study. A fuller description of the methodology affords other investigators the opportunity to repeat a study. Investigators who used multiple sites and international arenas supported the view that caring concerns are not setting-specific.

Despite the various methodologies used to explore caring within educational settings, common themes did emerge. Respect, being present, having competence, and fostering growth were some of these commonly identified themes. Students, faculty, and practicing nurses had similar definitions of caring. Faculty and students identified common frustrations that occurred when attempts were made to act in a more caring manner. Students, in particular, could identify uncaring behaviors that had been directed toward them. Perhaps the concept of caring is not as elusive as Morse, Solber, Neander, Bottorff, and Johnson (1990) suggested.

FUTURE DIRECTIONS

A body of research has emerged to illuminate how the curriculum revolution has helped to raise the awareness of caring concerns within educational programs in nursing. The majority of the completed research has dealt with students' definitions of caring and their perceptions of caring interactions with their instructors. To gain a deeper understanding of how nursing curricula are being transformed, more exploration of faculty perceptions of caring interactions with their students needs to be done. Diekelmann's (1990) narratives of dialogues with faculty should help in this regard. Perhaps a study similar to Benner's (1984) could help in our efforts to make curricula more caring. Faculty at various points in their careers could describe paradigm cases where caring occurred within educational environments. This same methodology, as well as other modes of inquiry, could be used for further study of students in the various nursing educational programs, to determine whether caring is defined and experienced differently in associate degree, diploma, baccalaureate, master's, and doctoral programs. Findings from studies such as Berman (1988), Eriksson (1989), and Chipman (1991) suggest, however, that caring is defined similarly across all programs.

Ethnographic studies like Berman's (1988) could further demonstrate how students and faculty conduct their lives within the nursing curriculum. Interviews are useful tools for gaining an understanding of perceptions of caring within educational environments. However, direct observations can help to verify and give additional insight into the nature of the settings where curricula are carried out.

Finally, more research needs to be done in which outcomes are investigated. If caring content is in the curriculum and caring practices take place within that curriculum, do graduates from the various nursing programs (associate degree, baccalaureate, master's, and doctoral) practice caring behaviors within the practice setting? Further, do these graduates practice caring differently? More long-term follow-up of graduates will shed light on whether transformation of the curriculum makes a difference in the patient care that is delivered by graduates from programs where those caring curriculum practices take place.

REFERENCES

Appleton, C. (1990). The meaning of human care and the experience of caring in a university school of nursing. In M. Leininger & J. Watson (Eds.), *The caring imperative in education* (pp. 77–93). New York: National League for Nursing.

Bauer, J. A. (1990). Caring as the central focus in nursing curriculum development. In M. Leininger & J. Watson (Eds.), *The caring imperative in education* (pp. 255–266). New York: National League for Nursing.

Beck, C. T. (1991). How students perceive faculty caring: A phenomenological study. *Nurse Educator, 16*(5), 18–22.

Benner, P. (1984). *From novice to expert: Excellence and power in clinical practice.* Menlo Park, CA: Addison-Wesley.

Berman, L. (1988). Dilemmas in teaching caring: An "outsider's" perspective. *Nursing Connections, 1*(3), 5–15.

Bevis, E. (1988). New directions for a new age. In *Curriculum revolution: Mandate for change* (pp. 27–52). New York: National League for Nursing.

Bevis, E. O., & Watson, J. (1989). *Toward a caring curriculum: A new pedagogy for nursing.* New York: National League for Nursing.

Carkhuff, R. N. (1969). *Helping and human relations, vol. 1.* New York: Holt, Rinehart and Winston.

Chipman, Y. (1991). Caring: Its meaning and place in the practice of nursing. *Journal of Nursing Education, 30,* 171–175.

Colaizzi, P. F. (1978). Psychological research as the phenomenologist views it. In R. Valle & M. King (Eds.), *Existential–phenomenological alternatives for psychology.* New York: Oxford University Press.

de Tornay, (1990). The curriculum revolution. *Journal of Nursing, 29,* 292–294.

Diekelmann, N. L. (1989). The nursing curriculum: Lived experiences of students. In *Curriculum revolution: Reconceptualizing nursing education* (pp. 25–41). New York: National League for Nursing.

Diekelmann, N. (1990). Nursing education: Caring, dialogue, and practice. *Journal of Nursing Education, 29,* 300–305.

Diekelmann, N. (1991). The emancipatory power of the narrative. In R. Schaperow (Ed.), *Curriculum revolution: Community building and activism* (pp. 41–62). New York: National League for Nursing.

Eriksson, K. (1989). Caring paradigms: A study of the origins and development of caring paradigms among nursing students. *Scandinavian Journal of Caring Sciences, 3,* 169–176.

Forsyth, D., Delaney, C., Maloney, N., Kubesh, D., & Story, D. (1989). Can caring behavior be taught? *Nursing Outlook, 37,* 164–166.

Friedrich, R. M., Lively, S. I., & Schacht, E. (1985). Teaching curriculum skills in an integrated curriculum. *Journal of Nursing Education, 24,* 164–166.

Giorgi, A. (1985). *Phenomenology and psychological research.* Pittsburgh: Duquesne University Press.

Glaser, B., & Strauss, A. (1973). *The discovery of grounded theory: Strategies for qualitative research.* Chicago: Aldine.

Halldorsdottir, S. (1990). The essential structure of a caring and uncaring encounter with a teacher: The perspective of the nursing student. In M. Leininger & J. Watson (Eds.). *The caring imperative in education* (pp. 95–107). New York: National League for Nursing.

Hughes, L. (1992). Faculty–student interactions and the student-perceived climate for caring. *Advances in Nursing Science, 14*(3), 60–71.

Kelly, B. (1990). Respect and caring: Ethics and essence in nursing. In M. Leininger (Ed.), *Ethical and moral dimensions of care* (pp. 67–79). Detroit: Wayne State University Press.

Kelly, B. (1991). The professional values of English nursing undergraduates. *Journal of Advanced Nursing, 16,* 867–872.

Kelly, B. (1992a). Professional ethics as perceived by American nursing undergraduates. *Journal of Advanced Nursing, 17,* 10–15.

Kelly, B. (1992b). The professional self-concept of nursing undergraduates and their perceptions of influential forces. *Journal of Nursing Education, 31,* 121–125.

Kersten, J., Bakewell, K., & Meyer, D. (1991). Motivating factors in a student's choice of nursing as a career. *Journal of Nursing Education, 30,* 30–33.

Komorita, N. I., Doehring, K. M., & Hirchert, P. W. (1991). Perceptions of caring by nurse educators. *Journal of Nursing Education, 30,* 23–29.

Kuhn, T. S. (1970). *The structure of scientific revolutions* (2nd ed.). Chicago, IL: University of Chicago Press.

LaMonica, E. L. (1983). Empathy can be learned. *Nurse Educator, 8,* (9), 19–23.

Lincoln, Y., & Guba, E. (1985). *Naturalistic inquiry.* Beverly Hills, CA: Sage.

Mangold, A. M. (1991). Senior nursing students' and professional nurses' perceptions of effective caring behaviors: A comparative study. *Journal of Nursing Education, 30,* 134–139.

Mangum, S., Garrison, C., Lind, C., Thackery, R., & Wyatt, M. (1991). Perceptions of nurses' uniforms. *Image: The Journal of Nursing Scholarship, 23,* 127–130.

Miller, B., Haber, J., & Byrne, M. W. (1990). The experience of caring in the teaching–learning process of nursing education: Student and teacher perspectives. In M. Leininger & J. Watson (Eds.), *The caring imperative in education* (pp. 125–135), New York: National League for Nursing.

Moccia, P. (1988). Curriculum revolution: An agenda for change. In *Curriculum revolution: Mandate for change* (pp. 53–64). New York: National League for Nursing.

Morse, J. M. (Ed.). (1991). *Qualitative nursing research: A contemporary dialogue.* Beverly Hills, CA: Sage.

Morse, J. M., Solber, S. M., Neander, W. L., Bottorff, J. L., & Johnson, J. L. (1990). Concepts of caring and caring as a concept. *Advances in Nursing Science, 13*(1), 1–14.

Nelms, T. P. (1990). The lived experience of nursing education: A phenomenological study. In M. Leininger & J. Watson (Eds.), *The caring imperative in education* (pp. 285–297). New York: National League for Nursing.

Noddings, N. (1988). An ethic of caring and its implications for instructional arrangements. *American Journal of Education, 96,* 215–230.

Norris, J. (1986). Teaching communication skills: Effects of two methods of instruction and selected learner characteristics. *Journal of Nursing Education, 25,* 102–106.

Pagana, K. D. (1988). Stresses and threats reported by baccalaureate students in relation to an initial clinical experience. *Journal of Nursing Education, 27,* 418–424.

Ray, M. (1987). Technological caring: A model in critical care. *Dimensions of Critical Care Nursing, 6,* 166–173.

Roach, Sr. S. (1984). *Caring: The human mode of being. Implications for nursing.* Perspectives in Caring Monograph No. 1. Toronto: University of Toronto Faculty of Nursing.

Rogers, I. A. (1986). The effects of undergraduate nursing education on empathy. *Western Journal of Nursing Research, 8,* 329–343.

Sheston, M. L. (1990). Caring in nursing education: A theoretical blueprint. In M. Leininger & J. Watson (Eds.), *The caring imperative in education* (pp. 109–123). New York: National League for Nursing.

Slevin, A. P., & Harper, M. O. (1987). The teaching of caring: A survey report. *Nurse Educator, 12*(6), 23–26.

Stephenson, P. M. (1984). Aspects of the nurse tutor–student nurse relationship. *Journal of Advanced Nursing, 9,* 283–290.

Tanner, C. A. (1990a). Caring as a value in nursing education. *Nursing Outlook, 38,* 70–72.

Tanner, C. A. (1990b). Reflections on the curriculum revolution. *Journal of Nursing Education, 29,* 295–299.

Theis, E. T. (1986). Nursing students' perspectives of unethical teaching behaviors. *Journal of Nursing Education, 27,* 102–106.

Watson, J. (1990). Caring knowledge and informed moral passion. *Advances in Nursing Science, 13*(1), 15–24.

Chapter Three

DOCTORAL EDUCATION IN NURSING: A COMPREHENSIVE REVIEW OF THE RESEARCH AND THEORETICAL LITERATURE

Sharon Hudacek, EdD, RN
Dona Marie Carpenter, EdD, RN

INTRODUCTION

Many routes exist for nurses to attain doctoral education. To members of the profession, selecting the degree that offers the most appropriate preparation for career goals is often puzzling and frustrating. The increasing number of programs and the different types of degrees offered make it more difficult for faculty to suggest to prospective students which program would best suit their educational needs.

Much of the recent literature suggests that doctoral education in nursing is moving toward a specific model and/or degree requirement. Debates within the profession now focus on quality, similarities, and differences in doctoral nursing education.

This chapter reviews and critiques research studies and theoretical literature addressing doctoral education in nursing. The Cumulative Index of Nursing and Allied Health Literature (CINAHL) was referenced, using the descriptors doctoral, nursing, and education. Bibliographies of several investigations were used to expand the review. Table 1 reviews the literature referenced in the paper.

Major questions and concerns in the review include: What has been learned throughout the 90-year history of doctoral education? Does diversity exist in doctoral education? How are doctoral programs the same, and how are they different? How has the quality of doctoral education in nursing been affected by the different types of programs and the increasing number of programs? What is the real need for nurses with doctoral degrees? What are the future directions and research agendas related to doctoral education in nursing?

Table 1. Chronological Outline of Nursing Studies Reviewed

Study	Date	Discussion/Purpose	Recommendations/Results
Elkins	1960	Caution to nursing regarding implementation of doctoral education.	Nursing was not ready for the doctorate, needed more clarity in goals and objectives for this degree.
McManus	1960	Rebuttal to Elkins (1960).	Nursing cannot afford *not* to develop doctoral programs.
Editorial	1963	Awarding of Boston University's first doctorate.	First DNS degree earned by a midwife, who had a major in psychiatric nursing.
Cleino	1965	Surveyed faculty member regarding educational background.	Actual interest in nursing education existed; 50 percent of those surveyed were actively engaged in research.
Kemble	1966	Review of the PhD route for doctoral education.	PhD recommended by author due to flexibility and consistency.
Hassenplug	1966	Questioned whether a theory existed for nursing science that would make possible the development of a PhD in nursing.	Suggested that nurses should enroll in established programs in natural or social sciences until substantial content in nursing was defined.
Nahm	1966	Addressed issue of doctoral education for the purpose of advancing nursing's clinical status.	Author supported the clinical doctorate with a strong emphasis on research and physical assessment skills.
Abdellah	1966	Analyzed differences between PhD and DNS degrees in an effort to define the "perfect" route to doctoral education.	Nursing needs both researcher and expert practitioners—currently, no "perfect" route.
Schlotfeldt	1966	Theoretical paper discussing the PhD focus for nursing.	PhD degree should be in a field of fundamental knowledge such as biology or psychology.
Peplau	1966	Two doctoral degrees exist for nurses—the DNSc and the PhD.	Advocated a dual degree route but emphasized that both degrees should be different.
Rogers	1966	Discussion of doctoral education in nursing and PhD.	Future directions of doctorally prepared nurses presented—focus on theoretical and applied research.

Taylor, Gifford, & Vian	1971	Studied characteristics in doctoral education.	PhD was a growing trend. Degree holders were predominantly being utilized in nursing education, service, and research.
Matarazzo & Abdellah	1971	Changing educational patterns in doctoral education, and influences of federal government.	Statistics reported on earned doctorates (1926–1970), support for doctoral education of USPHS (1956–1968), and future directions of nurse scientist degrees were reviewed.
Newman	1975	Supported a Doctor of Nursing degree.	Autonomy, independent practice will ensure professionalism.
Pitel & Vian	1975	Data collected for the international directory of nurses with doctoral degrees.	A trend for nurses to earn a PhD rather than EdD. Nurses earned doctoral degrees later in life but took no longer to complete degrees than doctorates in other fields.
Downs	1976	Examination of graduates' view of NYU, 1964–1974	All areas were viewed positively—the 81 respondents were involved in research and scholarly activity.
Cleland	1976	Discussion of the professional doctorate with three years of clinical specialization.	The author's model emphasized expert clinical practice with use of nursing research.
Leininger	1976	Overview of doctoral education in the United States—focus on trends, questions, and projections for the future.	Additional quality doctoral programs are needed, as well as doctorally prepared faculty. A need for federal, state, and private funds exists.
Christman	1978	Addressed issue of doctoral education for the purpose of advancing nursing's clinical status.	Author supported the clinical doctorate with a strong emphasis on research and physical assessment skills.
Downs	1978	Analysis of future directions in doctoral nursing education.	Upsurge in admissions in doctoral programs. Emphasis on quality rather than quantity programs.
Grace	1978	Historical development of nursing education.	History of "types of doctoral programs in nursing," EdD, DNS, PhD. Proposed models for development of doctoral programs in nursing.
Schlotfeldt	1978	The Doctor of Nursing degree.	Goal—hasten nursing's professional development toward a fully autonomous scholarly discipline.
Parietti	1979	Historical analyses of significant factors responsible for the development of doctoral education for nurses.	Doctoral education must maintain diversity and is critical in the preparation of future educators, researchers, and administrators.

Table 1. (*Continued*)

Study	Date	Discussion/Purpose	Recommendations/Results
Gorney-Fadiman	1981	Review of education doctorates, philosophy doctorates, and nonnursing PhDs.	Choice of degree to best support nursing employment is the PhD, from the authors' perspective/opinion.
Beare, Gray, & Ptak	1981	To identify essential content in doctoral programs.	Foci of doctoral curricula investigated: defending a theory base for nursing, changing health care delivery, funding needs, improving nursing image, and ethical issues.
Murphy	1981	To identify essential content in doctoral programs.	Functional specialists, nurse scientists, PhDs were presented. Conclusion that little consensus exists as to the scientific knowledge base of nursing at the doctoral level.
Curran, Habeeb, & Sobol	1981	Discussion of dilemma of selecting a doctoral program, given variety of programs existing.	Differences in programs unclear. Authors view ND as the only practice degree. PhD and EdD are well-established, DNS is not.
Perry	1982	Analysis of faculty teaching in doctoral nursing programs.	Majority of faculty do not possess academic credentials nor do they engage in scholarly research.
Brimmer, et al.	1983	Education and employment characteristics of nurses with doctoral degrees.	Nurses with doctorates were hired in their first positions as teachers, shifted to administrative roles in academia later in their careers.
Murphy	1984	Discussion of faculty as resources in the development of quality doctoral programs.	Faculty need to inform themselves continually of scholarship and research.
Murphy	1985	Literature review of doctoral education from 1950 to 1980.	Trends identified in doctoral education included: increases in graduates and programs, preference of PhD over EdD, and an increasing concern for research productivity.
Brown	1985	Theoretical review of types of doctoral programs available, trends in doctoral nursing education, and the need for doctorally prepared nurses.	Although a case was made for the non-nursing doctorates, the author suggested that the trend was toward the PhD in order to legitimize the profession.

Amos	1985	Quality issues in doctoral education.	Concern over large growth of doctoral programs, needs for doctorally prepared nurses, the nature of degrees, and the qualifications of students, as well as the overall program of study.
Loomis	1985	To describe the distribution of content in doctoral nursing education from 1976 to 1982.	In analyzing dissertation abstracts, 78.4 percent were clinical studies and 21.6 percent were social issue studies.
Lutz & Schlotfeldt	1985	Evaluation of the ND program at Case Western University. Philosophy and curriculum organization are addressed.	The program is worthwhile and expectations are that, in the near future, all nursing professionals will be prepared at the doctoral level.
Norris	1985	Review of a five-year projection in starting a doctoral nursing program.	Various needs of a new program: upgraded faculty, improved research, growth of theory and science of nursing, and acceptance in academia.
Anderson, Roth, & Palmer	1985	A national survey to document the need for doctoral programs in nursing.	A substantial need was documented for doctorally prepared nurses in both academic and health service areas. Expansion of doctoral programs was recommended.
Snyder-Halpern	1986	To clarify distinctions between research-oriented (PhD) and professionally oriented (DNSc) doctoral programs in nursing.	Similarities in outcome variables and curricular content. Both programs prepared educators and applied researchers; however, DNSc geared to the preparation of clinicians.
Brodie	1986	To investigate the impact of doctoral programs on nursing education.	Four major issues developed: (1) need/number of doctorally prepared nurses, (2) research, (3) faculty scholarly activity, and (4) faculty–university contributions.
Fitzpatrick, Kluznik–Boyle, & Anderson	1986	To evaluate the ND degree on performance of initial careers of ND and BSN program graduates.	Similar initial employment characteristics. Differences in graduate education and employment patterns, with ND grads progressing more rapidly in nontraditional roles.
Shores	1986	Analysis of decisions to initiate doctoral programs; 25 programs that offered a DNS or PhD degree were analyzed.	Recommendations included giving priority to hiring highly qualified faculty: doctorally prepared, with research abilities, teaching mastery, and proficiency in field of clinical expertise.

Table 1. (*Continued*)

Study	Date	Discussion/Purpose	Recommendations/Results
Andreoli	1986	PhD is the more popular degree.	Proposed a combination degree—the DNS/PhD model.
Holzemer & Chambers	1986	Examined the relationship between perceptions of the environment and scholarly productivity of both faculty and alumni of nursing doctoral programs.	Faculty and alumni research productivity was high when resources and support were perceived as readily available.
Holzemer	1987	Analysis of the growth and change in the quality of doctoral education from 1979 to 1984.	Despite the increase in doctoral programs, quality is not in jeopardy.
Seitz	1987	The pros and cons of doctoral education, in the author's opinion, are reviewed.	Pros: Creditability, advance and maintain quality of nursing profession. Cons: Expensive, narrow fields of study.
Edens & Labadie	1987	Discussion of the ND degree as a postbaccalaureate opinion.	ND was more attractive to individuals seeking late entry into the nursing profession, although concern exists over the impact of the ND on existing doctoral structure.
Lash	1987a	Competing philosophies in doctoral education in nursing.	Nursing should modify PhD model to fit goals of nursing.
Lash	1987b	Discussion of differences in doctoral education.	A lack of differentiation existed between preparation for academic and advanced clinical routes.
Werley & Leske	1988	Expanded review of literature on history and differences in doctoral programs.	Differing criteria are needed for PhD and DNS programs in order to set the direction of nursing's future.
Fields	1988	Discussion of types of doctoral programs. Historical review of literature.	The author reviews the PhD as the ultimate degree for most nurses and provides rationale.
Meleis	1988	Review of issues in doctoral education.	Societal trends, professional research degrees, history, faculty, and quality indicators are reported.
Downs	1988	Raised the issue of quality in view of the rapid expansion of doctoral programs.	Author not in favor of structure, criteria, and standards, and emphasized the need for high-quality peer culture participation.

VanDongen	1988	Phenomenological investigation of the life experience of full-time doctoral students.	Doctoral education significantly impacts on the personal life of the student, resulting in stress, restriction of social life, and intense concentration on education goals.
Blancett	1989	Editorial on differentiating doctoral degrees.	Review of 1989 AACN conference proceedings and emphasis on quality.
Williams	1989	Theoretical discussion of the relationship between the area of study concentration and focus of inquiry and the area of employment following doctoral education.	Individuals must be well-prepared in doctoral programs to develop clinical research or they will not be in demand, particularly in more competitive environments.
Anderson	1989	Discussed the issue of quality in doctoral education versus degree type.	Students must be prepared to do research that improves practice and disseminates research findings.
Forni	1989	Analysis of history of doctoral programs and types of programs in existence today.	The PhD was viewed as the degree "in the lead" in nursing.
Casarett	1989	To identify components needed to support graduate education.	Faculty involvement, research, formal instruction, process, and governance were several outcomes identified.
Wiley	1989	To analyze topics of dissertations in PhD programs.	The majority of topics were in nursing administration and theory/philosophical topics. Only 19 percent were clinical nursing topics.
Grace	1989	Issues in doctoral education.	Three types of degrees needed: (1) research doctoral, (2) clinical/applied research doctorate, and (3) professional doctorate.
Zebelman & Olswang	1989	To determine how many doctoral students in nursing identified the goal of "faculty" at the beginning of and 1 year after doctoral studies.	Career goals of doctoral nursing students change over time. More experienced students became less interested in faculty positions. EdD students were most interested in faculty positions.
Downs	1989	Differences between the professional doctorate and the academic/research doctorate.	A one-on-one fit may never be suitable in nursing, that is, in terms of one program for all students.
Bremner et al.	1990	Report on a survey concerning the number of doctorally prepared nursing vs. non-nursing	The number of nursing rather than non-nursing doctorates is increasing. A policy regarding an institution specifically

Table 1. (*Continued*)

Study	Date	Discussion/Purpose	Recommendations/Results
		faculty and the institutional requirements of a doctorate as the terminal degree.	requiring a "nursing doctorate" was not found in one-half of the respondents surveyed.
Marriner-Tomey	1990	To analyze the historical development of doctoral programs.	History of doctoral education was presented from the Middle Ages to current time.
Ketefian	1991	Discussed strategies that doctoral programs can use to better prepare students for their careers.	Role modeling by faculty was viewed as essential, along with goal setting to ease conflicting demands.
Gortner	1991	Reviewed the history of doctoral education in the United States.	Greater research emphasis on fundamental processes is needed, along with cross-disciplinary training in a revised nurse scientist model.
Farren	1991	To examine differences in research productivity of nurse doctorate.	No relationship was found between dissertation topic and postdoctoral research. Research support determined productivity.
Fitzpatrick	1991	Presentation of doctoral preparation versus expectations.	Twelve strategies were proposed to assist faculty in academia.
Barnum	1991	Discussion of doctoral education for nurse executives.	Advice to nurse executives was offered related to doctoral education available to nurses in this role.
Ziemer et al.	1992	Review of curriculum and philosophy based on catalogue descriptions of programs.	More similarities than differences exist in doctoral education.

REVIEW OF THE LITERATURE: HISTORICAL EVOLUTION

The doctorate as an earned degree originated in Europe during the Middle Ages. Yale University had the distinction, in 1861, of being the first American institution to award the Doctor of Philosophy degree (Matarazzo & Abdellah, 1971). Nearly 60 years later, the first doctorate in nursing was available.

Many factors were responsible for the development of doctoral education for nurses; among those most significant were the industrialization of the nation, pressures of war, demand by the public for higher education, and the feminist movement. Doctoral education was viewed as critical in the preparation of future educators, researchers, and administrators, and continues to be so today (Parietti, 1979).

The first doctoral program specifically for nurses was developed in 1899 at Teachers College, Columbia University, New York (Grace, 1978). Graduates of Teachers College earned the EdD (Doctor of Education), which prepared teachers and administrators as functional specialists. Teachers College was at the forefront of nursing education and designed a program that focused on both the educational and nursing needs of leaders in the profession. "Teachers College is the only American institution to combine a nursing and education degree, in the form of two programs: in curriculum and nursing instruction, and in administration of education" (Gorney-Fadiman, 1981, p. 662).

In 1934, New York University became the second institution to offer a doctoral degree in nursing. Graduates earned a PhD (Doctor of Philosophy). The University of Pittsburgh followed in the 1950s. The PhD is considered a research-oriented degree that prepares nurses for intellectual inquiry that will develop the science of nursing practice (Werley & Leske, 1988).

As doctoral education in nursing emerged, differences of opinion arose. The nursing profession was cautioned to be very precise and careful in implementing doctoral education. In the early 1960s, the goals and objectives of the nursing doctorate had not been clearly delineated. Little agreement existed among nursing leaders on the topic in 1960. More deliberation and critical consideration of all aspects of program development were required (Elkins, 1960).

McManus (1960) offered a rebuttal to Elkins's writings. She believed that nursing was obligated to develop programs in doctoral education and could not afford not to. Further, she argued that nursing needed to create new knowledge through basic research on the doctoral level.

Another barrier to doctoral education in nursing during the 1960s was the fact that a theoretical framework for nursing science remained unclear. It was suggested that nurses enroll in established programs in the natural and social sciences until substantive content in nursing was defined (Hassenplug, 1966).

Kemble (1966) believed that it was appropriate to follow the PhD route. She was not in favor of adding other titles to doctoral programs studied by nurses. Further, Kemble emphasized that the PhD is an "open-ended degree, which permits flexibility in planning the program of studies" (p. 43).

The historical development of the PhD was analyzed by Lash (1987). According to Lash, the PhD should present a free spirit of inquiry by being a teaching doctorate and a literary doctorate that demonstrates scholarship (p. 97). Lash believed the PhD would accommodate the practice concerns of nursing because it is both broad and specialized. Nursing should "modify the PhD model in ways to improve the fit between the goals of nursing and the degree" (p. 100).

During the 1970s, the professional practice doctorate was promoted as the terminal degree for nursing. Newman (1975) believed that the four-year baccalaureate degree was not sufficient to prepare a nurse for the "independent practice" of nursing needed by consumers of health care. Newman focused on the concepts of autonomy and independent practice, promoting the professional doctorate—the doctorate of nursing science—as the means to an advanced educational base and improved professional status.

Taylor, Gifford, and Vian (1971) analyzed information, collected for the American Nurses Foundation's Directory of Nurses, on nurses who had earned doctorates. The study population consisted of 587 nurses with doctorates. Data collection included numerous variables—field of doctoral study, degree type, university, present position and responsibility, employer and clinical interest. Of those studied, 90 percent were clearly involved in nursing. Four-fifths of the sample were employed as faculty members in educational institutions, and almost 40 percent held administrative positions in their institutions. Sixty percent were working in 47 schools that offered graduate degrees. One-third of all respondents were actively engaged in research. An educational trend was noted among the types of degree earned. In the 1960s, the EdD dominated; in the 1970s, the

PhD appeared to increase in popularity. Employment characteristics revealed that the majority of nurses were working full-time in nursing education, service, and research.

Pitel and Vian (1975) used the same study design used by Taylor, Gifford, and Vian (1971) but added foreign countries to their inquiry. Survey data elicited a number of trends: (1) the Doctor of Philosophy degree (PhD) was becoming the preferred degree for nurses; (2) the educational progression from post-high school to the doctorate lacked articulation; and (3) the time span required to complete the doctorate for nurses was no longer than the degree time in other disciplines. The Doctor of Education (EdD) was the major type of doctoral degree granted in the 1950s, and the PhD and the Doctor of Nursing Science (DNSc) were the degrees most often awarded in the 1960s and 1970s. Numerous other demographic findings were reported, such as age, clinical specialty, employment profile, and locations of doctoral institutions.

According to Murphy (1981), doctoral education for nursing evolved in three phases. In phase one (1926–1959), nurses emerged as functional specialists. During this phase, the majority of doctorates were in education, and nurses were prepared as teachers and administrators. This phase reflected nursing's first efforts at doctoral education for the profession (Murphy, 1981).

In phase two (1960–1969), nurses graduated as nurse scientists. Nurses were now beginning to seek both nursing and non-nursing doctorates. Program choice also increased as the number of doctoral programs available to nurses grew. The need to prepare faculty to teach and the availability of research fellowships contributed to program growth. Issues that emerged during this second phase continue to impact on the evolution of doctoral education in nursing. They include: What is the essential nature of professional nursing? What is the substantive knowledge base of professional nursing? What kind of research is important for nursing as a knowledge discipline and as a practice discipline? How can the scientific base of nursing knowledge be identified and expanded? (Murphy, 1981, p. 646.)

The third phase of doctoral education in nursing began in 1971 when a committee of nursing leaders first gathered together to address the future of doctoral education nursing. The central issue for this discussion was what type or types of doctoral preparation should be recommended for the future. The recommendation for the PhD in nursing emerged from these discussions.

In another review, Matarazzo and Abdellah (1971) traced doctoral education in the United States from the founding of Harvard College in 1636 to the establishment of the first American PhD degree at Yale in 1861. Using the overall history of non-nursing doctoral education to support their discussion, the authors reported the history of doctoral education for nursing. Changing educational patterns from 1950 to 1970 were analyzed. Their discussion of the nursing doctorate compares the development of nursing with other disciplines such as the medical and engineering doctorates. The influence of the federal government in furthering the doctoral education of nurses was reviewed as was the research training support for nurse researchers.

Leininger (1976) surveyed doctoral programs in the United States with a focus on trends, questions, and projections for the future. Her questionnaire provided data on 30 variables; among them were new and established programs, by region and degree; nurse faculty; preferred doctoral degree; and financial support of doctoral programs. Findings indicated that, of the established and future planned doctoral programs, 20 were offering the PhD, 11 the DNSc (or DN, or DNS), and 1 a PhD in health sciences. A 61 percent increase, from 1973 to 1976, was noted in doctorally prepared nurse faculty. Regarding the "preferred" doctorate, the majority of respondents (26 of 46) chose the PhD; 16 of 46 chose the DNS. Estimated financial support for doctoral programs indicated that almost all of the programs received insufficient state funding. Participants were asked to identify, in order of priority, the three greatest needs for preparation of nurses in doctoral study. These needs were identified: increased number of well-prepared faculty to teach and do nursing research in master's and doctoral programs; increased preparation of nurses as researchers; increased publication of nursing research studies; and institutional funds to support schools of nursing offering doctoral programs.

Perhaps one of the most comprehensive historical reviews on doctoral education in nursing was completed by Grace (1978). She discussed the profession's development prior to the late 1800s and up to the first graduate education available to nurses at Teacher's College, Columbia University, in the early 1900s. Historical studies of nursing education, such as the Goldmark Report, and federal funding sources were detailed. A critique of types of doctoral programs was presented. Future models for doctoral programs in nursing were considered. The ideal model, according to Grace (1978), would have a priority for the development of research, critical thinking, and analysis and synthesis of nursing theory.

The 1950s and 1960s were a time of great educational change, according to Marriner-Tomey (1990). National, regional, and governmental decisions about nursing education were reviewed. Studies described recent research that went beyond discussing types of programs and emphasized similarities and differences in programs. Based on this analysis, a trend toward the PhD as the doctoral degree for nurses was apparent.

After an extensive review of doctoral program history in nursing, including a focus on the student and the diversity of student characteristics, Gortner (1991) suggested that nursing should reexamine the nursing scientist model and maintain diversity in doctoral educational pathways.

In summary, most studies have focused on historical development of the doctorate in nursing, citing the phases of program development, program types, research, and theory needs. All studies were quantitative in nature and were designed to collect mostly demographic data about enrollment, completion time frames, and program characteristics over approximately 90 years of doctoral education. Trends noted in the historical literature included the PhD's gaining popularity; the increased number of doctorally prepared faculty teaching in doctoral education, particularly in the mid-1970s, and continued funding concerns for existing and future doctoral programs in nursing.

TYPES OF DOCTORAL PROGRAMS IN NURSING

Nurse scholars often are asked to distinguish among doctoral program types. Similarities and differences in EdD, PhD, DNS, and ND programs can be vast, and program selection should be grounded in familiarity with the program types.

American doctoral degrees are awarded in the arts and sciences; in traditional professions such as theology, medicine, and nursing; and in newer professional fields such as business administration, library science, and social work (Harris, Trout, & Andrews, 1980). The question of which is the appropriate doctoral degree has emerged in every discipline. Nursing has yet to reach a consensus on doctoral education (Grace, 1978). Perhaps the first step in resolving some of these issues is to identify the similarities and differences among the various types of programs (PhD, EdD, DNSc).

The literature suggests that similarities of doctoral programs far exceed differences. The broad requirements of all programs, no matter what the discipline, include: demonstration of mastery of a specific body of knowledge, demonstration of research skill, and design and completion of an original piece of research in one's area of specialization (Harris et al., 1980; Pitel & Vian, 1975).

Three types of doctorates are available to nurses seeking a terminal degree: Doctor of Education (EdD), Doctor of Philosophy (PhD), and Doctor of Nursing Science (DNSc). In contemporary nursing literature, analysis of the varying nursing doctorates is offered by several authors (Anderson, 1989; Anderson, Roth, & Palmer, 1985; Barnum, 1991; Blancett, 1989; Brodie, 1986; Casarett, 1989; Seitz, 1987).

As noted earlier, the EdD was the most commonly awarded degree of the 1950s (Pitel & Vian, 1975). Members of the profession generally state that the EdD tends to be a pedagogical degree.

In the 1960s and 1970s, there was a trend toward attainment of the PhD (Fields, 1988). This degree has been identified as a research or academic degree.

The DNSc has been identified as a clinical research degree. Murphy (1981) emphasized that the focus of the DNS and DNSc is on expansion of the scientific knowledge base in clinical nursing. The federal government's program of research fellowship that supported the scientific basis of nursing provided the impetus for these programs. Boston University awarded its first doctorate in nursing science (DNS) in 1963 to a Kentucky midwife (Boston's first, 1963). The Boston doctoral program was initiated in 1960, with all students majoring in psychiatric nursing. A balance in academic and clinical activities was the intent of the program, which focused on treating "various mental illnesses" (p. 27).

Schlotfeldt (1966) noted that the PhD degree was most suitable for scholarly nurses. The contribution of Schlotfeldt's thinking was her belief that the PhD degree should be in a field of "fundamental knowledge" (p. 69), which included biology, psychology, or a similar subspecialty such as history—particularly if nursing history was the focus of study. Her premise was that a nurse pursuing a doctoral education degree could not be scholarly in the many areas applicable to nursing practice.

Schlotfeldt went on to develop the program of professional nursing study leading to the Doctor of Nursing (DN) in 1979 at Case Western University. This approach to preparing registered nurses focused on entry into practice at the doctoral level. The need to

(1) hasten nursing's professional development toward a fully autonomous scholarly discipline and (2) reorient nursing's approach to the preparation of professionals were primary objectives (Schlotfeldt, 1978). Students with graduate and undergraduate degrees in natural and behavioral sciences composed the majority of the student admissions in ND programs. Graduate follow-up studies indicated that 78 percent of the graduates were employed in acute care settings and several had gone on to medical school (Lutz & Schlotfeldt, 1985).

Fitzpatrick, Kluznik-Boyle, and Anderson (1986), in a graduate follow-up study, noted that NDs progressed at a more rapid pace than BSN graduates. ND graduates also sought more nontraditional roles than nurses with generic BSNs. Although outcome data of graduates are positive and national support for the ND exists, there is concern over the impact the ND may have on current doctoral education (Edens & Labadie, 1987).

DOCTORAL EDUCATION IN NURSING—SIMILARITIES OR DIFFERENCES?

Historically, nurse leaders have debated the issue of doctoral education in nursing and have searched, in varying ways, for answers about program diversity. The research and scholarly opinions of leaders in the profession follow.

Rogers (1966) emphasized that nursing is in need of philosophers who have knowledge of physics. She advocated nursing science as the core of the PhD program, with doctoral students building knowledge in logic and theory and possessing a strong background in math, statistics, and research design. Humanities and the natural and social sciences must be cognate courses. Finally, the major in doctoral education should be *nursing,* not higher education or related fields such as philosophy, education, or psychology.

Peplau (1966) believed two doctoral degrees existed for nurses: (1) the DNSc or expert practitioner, and (2) the PhD, with emphasis on theory and the production of original new knowledge. In the mid-1960s, Peplau advocated this dual degree route, emphasizing that both degrees are appropriate but each is different. "The difference is one of emphasis in the educational program" (p. 66). The DNSc emphasizes practice; the PhD emphasizes research.

Citing little need for a program title, Nahm (1966) stated that what is truly important is the use of nursing's prior knowledge to "verify what is known and elucidate what is not known" (p. 38). The doctorate should be the beginning of a search for knowledge and should develop leaders. Advanced preparation for nurses is the most important factor.

In the 1960s, little consensus existed in defining the perfect route for doctoral education. Nursing was in need of both researchers and expert practitioners in doctoral education. The PhD was viewed as providing depth in research, and the DNS as providing breadth of preparation in a clinical field.

Abdellah (1966) noted that there was no consensus in defining the route for doctoral education, and that nursing needs researchers and expert practitioners. Abdellah analyzed the terms "depth" and "breadth" in doctoral education as follows: The PhD is for those wishing depth in pursuing research, and the DNS is a route for breadth of preparation in a clinical field (p. 50).

Cleland (1976) favored the development of a postbaccalaureate generic professional program with three years of clinical specialization. Examples of this professional degree include the DNSc, Doctor of Public Health (DPH), and EdD. In Cleland's view, the professional doctorate model was compatible with American society and would allow for nursing to be recognized in patient care management. The primary focus of Cleland's model was on expert clinical practice rather than research/investigation, although she believed graduates needed to use research.

Christman (1978) favored enhancement of nursing's clinical status at the doctoral level. "Nurses must begin to compare their clinical posture with that of other clinicians [such as dentists]" (p. 45). Christman supported the clinical doctorate with a strong emphasis on research and physical assessment skills.

To clarify distinctions between PhD and DNS doctoral programs in nursing, Snyder-Halpern (1986) studied four programs of each type in order to evaluate curricular design and outcome variables. Close similarities were found in curricular content, suggesting that both program types are geared toward preparing educators and applied researchers. One difference noted was in the preparation of clinicians: DNS programs were more geared to the preparation of clinicians, whereas PhD programs tended to be more oriented to the preparation of pure researchers. In addition, DNS programs were considered more flexible in program structure and less traditional in teaching strategies. Snyder-Halpern suggested that true diversity is present in our emerging doctoral pathways.

Beare, Gray, and Ptak (1981) used a descriptive study to identify similarities in content in 12 doctoral programs in nursing. Similar content in all doctoral nursing programs included nursing theory, theory development, concept formulation, and quantitative analysis. Several authors have noted similar viewpoints (Fields, 1988; Gorney-Fadiman, 1981; Meleis, 1988).

Brown (1985) supported the PhD in nursing. "Most people recognize the PhD as the ultimate educational credential; nursing doctorate programs need to offer the PhD" (p. 20). "Doctorates outside of nursing do not promote the discipline. Nursing research and nursing theory development would advance the profession (p. 20)."

Forni (1989) also recognized the PhD as the primary degree in nursing. She further indicated that two basic models in nursing have emerged: (1) the PhD and (2) the DNS or DNSc degrees. The author espoused that, in reality, the distinction between degrees is not clear.

Downs (1989) reported statistical data comparing curricula in 43 DNS and PhD programs. DNS programs required an average of 21.37 clinical hours, and PhD programs had an average of only 3.52 clinical hours. She noted that it was impossible to define what clinical hours were, in many cases, in relation to the distribution of theory credits. DNSc programs had a mean of 13.87 credit hours and PhD programs had a mean of 15 to 30 credit hours. The mean of credit hours for research in DNS programs was 19.55; for the PhD programs, it was 25. The mean number of hours of statistics for the DNS was 12.75; for the PhD, it was 14.90. Overall, DNS programs have considerably more clinical time and PhD programs place more emphasis on statistics and research.

Grace (1989) suggested that differences should exist in doctoral programs. In support of Grace were several other authors who promoted this emerging concept of diversity (American Association of Colleges of Nursing's (AACN) Doctoral Conference, 1989; Downs, 1988; Moccia, 1986). Citing the field of psychology as an example, Grace noted that both experimental and clinical psychologists are accepted by the profession. By contrast, she contended that nursing adopts the position that nurses should and can do all: research, practice, theory, leadership. Promoting diverse needs of doctoral education, the author recommended three models: (1) the research doctorate, (2) the clinical/applied doctorate, and (3) the professional doctorate. The research doctorate would develop the knowledge base of the discipline and would need to be a basic postgraduate program that focuses on research skills. The clinical/applied doctorate would build on a clinical specialist foundation to prepare advanced practitioners for such areas as clinical teaching and clinical research. The professional doctorate would build on a general education background of a baccalaureate and would provide education in clinical practice and knowledge needs for professional practice as a nurse. Degree titles such as PhD would be purposely avoided. Grace suggested that current programs fail to prepare either competent researchers or applied practitioners and that a dramatic change in our views of doctoral education is needed.

Dissertation abstracts were analyzed by Loomis (1985), who described the content of nursing doctoral program dissertations. When differences in dissertation content by type of degree program (PhD, EdD, and DNS) were studied, EdD programs had more dissertations examining developmental life changes and studied educational variables more than other programs did. DNS programs studied educational variables significantly more than PhD programs did. The PhD program dissertations were more frequently focused on cultural human response system variables (p. 117). No significant differences were found between degree type and clinical decision-making variables.

Wiley (1989) surveyed nursing schools that offered the PhD degree in nursing. Thirty-two deans were queried by letter on dissertation topics and categories of accepted research in their doctoral programs. Findings indicated that three foci were acceptable for a PhD: (1) clinical nursing (96 percent), (2) nursing administration (67 percent), and (3) nursing education (59 percent). Three deans cautioned that, in some cases, dissertations needed to fit faculty expertise.

Farren (1991) found that degree type influences research activity. In a study of 152 nurses with doctorates, degree type proved to be significantly related to research productivity. Nurses with the PhD (47 percent) and DNS degrees (42 percent) were in the top research-producing groups, followed by nurses with the EdD degree (18 percent). Ninety-six percent of all nurses surveyed felt competent to perform research investigations.

Andreoli (1986) stated that, "in the real world," a difference in degrees is not clear. Citing the PhD is the more popular degree and the DNS as an advanced clinical practice doctorate, Andreoli proposed a combination degree, the DNS/PhD model. She supported eliminating diversity and establishing consensus for what a doctorate in nursing should require. Moccia (1986) noted that none of the doctoral degrees was a nursing doctorate, but that each indicated "a particular approach/interest to a common content area" (p. 265).

Lash (1987b) stated that a lack of differentiation exists between preparation for academic and advanced clinical roles. She cited similarities between the lack of differentiation of basic nursing preparation and that noted in doctoral education. "It appears that history is about to repeat itself on the doctoral level" (p. 224). Lash summarized "rival conceptions" in doctoral nursing education and the outcomes of competing philosophies of nursing doctorates. These include multiple doctoral titles and undifferentiated curricula.

Meleis (1988) suggested that the DNS program should "slowly but surely be phased out to declare the PhD as the official degree of the future" (p. 44). The author noted that the profession "cannot live" with the diversity in degrees and that the PhD reflects current professional needs (p. 439).

Curran, Habeeb, and Sobol (1981) discussed the dilemma of selecting a doctoral program for a career in nursing, in view of the variety of programs that exists (PhD, EdD, DNS). The authors noted that differences in programs are just not clear. "A persistent myth identifies the DNS as a practice degree; however, the DNS does not propose to prepare clinical practitioners" (p. 27). The only practice doctorate, in the authors' viewpoint, is the ND program at Case Western Reserve University. A degree such as the PhD or EdD is well-established in academic communities; the DNS is not.

Philosophy, curricula, and program requirements for 44 doctoral nursing programs were examined by Zeimer et al. (1992). Thirty-one PhD programs, 11 DNS, and 1 EdD participated in the study. The authors found that more similarities than differences existed in programs, regardless of the degree awarded. Most programs were built on master's degrees in nursing and required 60 additional credits. The dissertation seminar required more credits in certain programs. The curricula in all doctoral programs reflected an emphasis on research competence, with a major focus on quantitative research methodologies (p. 60). The authors noted that the programs gave limited attention to data management, tools and technology, and the acquisition of foreign language skills (p. 61).

VanDongen (1988) used phenomenological methodology to investigate full-time doctoral students' perceptions of doctoral education. From the students' perspective, doctoral education prompted many life changes and experiences and focused intensely on educational goals, stress, and restriction of certain social life experiences.

Summary statements of the *Proceedings* from the American Association of Colleges of Nursing's 1989 Doctoral Conference addressed diversity in doctoral education as "valued" (Booth, 1989). Diversity

Table 2. Similarities and Differences of Doctoral Programs

Similarities	Differences
Attendance at lectures and seminars, and discussions	Practical problem or survey versus basic research study in areas of research interest
Independent study in area of interest/specialization	EdD: Examines developmental life changes
Research design and implementation that contributes to a specific body of knowledge	PhD: Examines physical human response systems
Completion of formal course work	PhD: Pure research
Comprehensive written and oral examinations	DnSc: Clinical role
Oral defense of research and dissertation	
Four to five years of study	
Residency requirement	
Empowerment	
Networking	
Scholarship	
Dissonance	

in the models of programs used was thought to be a positive position taken by the profession.

Research reported in both the nursing and non-nursing literature indicates that many similarities exist in doctoral education. Opinions of numerous nurse leaders are split: some offer suggestions for uniformity and standardization of one doctoral degree for the future; others fear that, if one degree is established, the richness of diversity will be sacrificed. The 1989 AACN Doctoral Conference *Proceedings* suggested growing support for diversity, as long as programs provide a substantial knowledge base for students who seek doctoral nursing education. Table 2 lists similarities and differences in doctoral programs.

QUALITY AND EXCELLENCE

Because of a rapid proliferation of programs, the quality of doctoral education in nursing is an ongoing issue. The increase in number of programs is related to nurses' growing interest in pursuing a doctorate. To date, 54 programs offer a doctoral degree in nursing. The rapid growth of doctoral programs has led many educators to be concerned about issues surrounding quality of doctoral programs, faculty excellence, and the need for doctorally prepared nurses (Bremner, Crutchfield, Kosowski, Perkins, & Williams, 1990; Brodie, 1986; Casarett, 1989). In fact, it would seem that the ultimate degree debate is centered around issues of quality rather than which letters appear after the graduates' names.

The growth of doctoral education has been viewed both positively and negatively by members of the profession. On the positive side, more programs to develop and test theory and invite research would only strengthen the knowledge base of the nursing profession. Issues that have the potential to negatively affect the quality of doctoral education include lack of prepared faculty, inadequate course work in research and fields of expertise, less competitive admission standards, and programmatically weak research agendas.

Downs (1976) reported on a study of 81 graduates of the doctoral nursing program at New York University from 1964 to 1974. The study was designed to elicit data about faculty competence, course content, and dissertation importance. The majority of respondents felt the dissertation was very important and fostered self-discipline and independence. Of the graduates surveyed, 57 were employed in academic institutions and the remainder worked in research or administrative settings. Since receiving their doctorate, 50 percent had completed research on topics such as pregnancy, biological rhythms, and aging. In addition, assessment of faculty competence was rated high (3.61 to 4.0, on a 4-point scale). Downs summarized the study by noting that doctoral graduates are very motivated in pursuing a difficult body of scientific knowledge.

In 1965, using mailed questionnaires, Cleino surveyed approximately 100 nurse faculty members with doctorates. Eighty-one of the 94 participants had majored in professional or nursing education, contrary to the belief that nurses in the 1960s studied in fields other than nursing. This study also demonstrated that an active interest in doctoral education existed. One-third of the participants had served as head of at least one major research project, and approximately half were actively engaged in research. The desire of nurse faculty to maintain scholarship in their field and to remain committed to an active research agenda was apparent.

Amos (1985) further elaborated on issues in doctoral preparation in nursing at the American Association of Colleges of Nursing's (AACN) Doctoral Conference. She summarized the following issues affecting quality in doctoral education: (1) the large growth of doctoral programs; (2) the increase in the number of graduates from doctoral programs; (3) the increased need for doctorally prepared nurses; (4) the nature of degrees; (5) the program of study; (6) the capabilities of schools of nursing; and (7) qualifications of students.

Murphy (1985) assessed quality in doctoral education in a literature review spanning the period from 1950 to 1980. Trends noted in doctoral education included an increase in nurses' completing their degrees; an increase in nursing programs offering doctorates; a preference for the PhD over the EdD; and an increased concern for research among doctoral faculty and students. The results of Murphy's review indicated that quality is improving in doctoral education, but actual research activity by nurses with earned doctorates is low.

Anderson (1989) stated that nursing education needs faculty who have an established track record in research and scholarship. The quality of doctoral preparation, not degree type, is the issue. Theoretical knowledge and research background are needed. Anderson further noted that, if doctoral students are to get a quality education, the major expectations of faculty should be (1) research that improves practice and (2) dissemination of research findings.

Downs (1988) raised the issue of quality, in view of the rapid expansion of doctoral programs. She documented serious concerns for the quality in doctoral education and the impact of substandard programs on the future of nursing. Downs reportedly disfavored strict criteria and standards for doctoral education and expressed an opinion that students should participate in a "peer culture" and should question rather than follow standards.

Holzemer (1987), an advocate for quality in nursing education, analyzed the growth and change in quality of doctoral education from 1979 to 1984. Fourteen doctoral programs participated in two evaluation projects, one in 1979 and the other in 1984. Data indicated strong faculty commitment to scholarly activities, including publication and presentation of research. Regarding student admission criteria, students who entered programs in 1984 had higher GPAs than those accepted in 1979. Students perceived a significantly better quality of teaching from 1979 to 1984.

Several authors noted that the quality of doctoral education is inconsistent. Enrollment needs, recruitment of qualified faculty, and program reputations have been cited as factors influencing the quality of education and research productivity in doctoral programs (Anderson, 1989; Downs, 1988).

Meleis (1988) wrote that programs are being implemented that lack the "ingredients" to merit scholarship. Meleis suggested that doctoral programs should be monitored by a "National Peer

Consulting Team." The team would consult with new programs and assess established programs, utilizing peer review.

A lack of faculty educated in research impacts on the quality of doctoral programs. Brodie (1986) emphasized that the "relentless pressure of academic life" is very difficult for most faculty (p. 353). The issues of tenure, promotion, and keeping abreast of clinical changes in nursing and medical science are all too demanding. Research, largely because it is expected, is becoming more of a priority than good teaching.

Many nursing faculty have not established research agendas. In this regard, how can they teach the research process if they have never lived it? Anderson (1989) wrote that it is expected that faculty are good teachers, but the faculty should "have ongoing, active programs of research in their laboratories" (p. 251). She also noted that many nursing faculty are not prepared in their doctoral programs to do research.

Holzemer and Chambers (1986) examined the relationship between perceptions of the environment and scholarly productivity of both faculty and alumni of doctoral nursing programs. When available resources (i.e., research support) were perceived as high by faculty, faculty productivity was high. This also was true with student commitment and motivation: if both were high, so was faculty productivity. In addition, when faculty held a higher rank (associate vs. assistant), the environment was perceived by students as more favorable. This research seems to support the notion that highly productive faculty are strongly supported by students and alumni. Students search for quality from seasoned faculty of high rank.

Fitzpatrick (1991) noted that inquiring, high-quality minds are vital in nursing education. In citing "ideal faculty," she stated that several key ingredients were necessary: background and familiarity with research and grantsmanship; clinical expertise; teaching mastery; and knowledge of curriculum. She also noted that mastery of teaching and research are, unfortunately, not characteristic of new faculty teaching in nursing education. It is often the responsibility of the employing institution to strengthen these characteristics in new doctorally prepared faculty.

Murphy (1984) wrote that faculty are an extremely essential resource for developing a quality doctoral program in nursing. Faculty need to inform themselves continually of scholarship and research, explore new knowledge, and commit to service and excellence (p. 7).

Shores (1986) analyzed decisions to initiate doctoral nursing programs by assessing 25 programs offering DNS and PhD degrees.

Table 3. Summary of Conferences on Doctoral Education

Conferences	Year	Location	Central Issues
First national conference on Doctoral Education in Nursing	June 23–24, 1977	University of Pennsylvania, Philadelphia	Historical review, faculty resources, qualifications for student admission, program design, course content, and financial resources.
Proceedings of the 1978 Forum on Doctoral Education in Nursing	June 29–30, 1978	Rush University, Chicago	The professional doctorate in nursing, the nurse science doctorate, the researcher doctorate, and programs in nursing.
Proceedings of the 1979 Forum on Doctoral Education in Nursing	June 29–30, 1979	Jack Tar Hotel, San Francisco	Clinical content of nursing, quality-in-nursing doctoral dissertations, doctoral program evaluation, preparing nursing doctorates to participate in the scientific community.
Fourth National Forum on Doctoral Education in Nursing	June 26–27, 1980	Wayne State University, Detroit	Patterning of human behavior, patterning of sleep and respirations during sleep, caring and caring life-style, program evaluation—in doctoral education.
Fifth National Forum on Doctoral Education in Nursing	June 25–26, 1981	University of Washington, Seattle	Structures for research productivity, competing themes of science, mentorship for scholarliness, programmatic structure for research productivity.
Sixth National Forum on Doctoral Education in Nursing	June 24–25, 1982	Case Western Reserve University, Cleveland	Substantive content in the sociocultural and biophysiological and psychosocial domains.
Seventh National Forum on Doctoral Education in Nursing	June 23–24, 1983	New York University, New York	Analysis of dissertation abstracts and titles, students' viewpoint, nursing research grants and part-time doctoral students; needs and strengths.
Proceedings 1984 National Forum on Doctoral Education	June 21–22, 1984	University of Colorado, Denver	The doctor of nursing science, the clinical doctorate, epistemological strategies

			in nursing, operationalization of quality dimensions in doctoral programs, postdoctoral training for research program development.
Ninth National Forum on Doctoral Education in Nursing	June 13–14, 1985	University of Alabama, Birmingham	What is health? Toward a theory of family health, healthy doctoral programs: (1) an administrative perspective, (2) faculty members' perspective, and (3) a doctoral students' perspective.
Proceedings of the 1986 National Forum on Doctoral Education in Nursing	June 11–13, 1986	University of California, San Francisco	Client environment interactions, feminism, knowledge development, methodological issues, analysis of faculty productivity, and student support.
Proceedings of the 1987 National Forum on Doctoral Education in Nursing	June 25–26, 1987	Sheraton Hotel, Pittsburgh, PA	Public policy, welfare policy, social welfare, community mental health.
Proceedings of the 1988 Forum on Doctoral Education in Nursing	June 15–17, 1988	Westin La Paloma, Tucson, AZ	History and philosophy of science, nursing science, philosophy of science in doctoral curricula.
Proceedings for the 1989 National Forum on Doctoral Education in Nursing	June 7–9, 1989	Holiday Inn, Indianapolis, IN	Conceptual bases for the organization and advancement of nursing knowledge: clinical content, metaparadigm domain concepts, nursing diagnosis/taxonomy.
Proceedings of the 1990 National Forum on Doctoral Education in Nursing	1990	University of Texas, Austin	Preparation of nursing scholars, alternative approaches to organizing and advancing nursing knowledge, alternative approaches to preparing nurse scholars, uniformity and diversity in doctoral programs.

A questionnaire provided descriptive data related to factors that impact on decisions to initiate doctoral programs. One major recommendation offered to schools of nursing considering doctoral program initiation focused on quality faculty: "Give first priority to securing adequate highly qualified faculty" (p. 29). To satisfy the need for quality faculty for a quality program, faculty members would need a doctorate and would be required to exhibit research abilities, teaching mastery, and current knowledge of their field of nursing.

Casarett (1989) noted that a "critical mass" of faculty (p. 256) is needed in doctoral education. Students need to be exposed to a variety of faculty who have different world views, experiences, and philosophies.

In summary, six indicators of the quality of doctoral programs for PhD, DNS, and EdD degrees in nursing have been endorsed by authorities in nursing (AACN Doctoral Conference, 1984): (1) faculty, (2) programs of study, (3) resources, (4) students, (5) research, and (6) evaluation criteria are documented in the literature as indicators of quality. In 1978, forums on doctoral education in nursing were initiated because of the expressed need of faculty members in established doctoral programs to exchange ideas. The conferences continue to this date. Table 3 summarizes the central issues and conclusions of these conferences.

THE NEED FOR DOCTORALLY PREPARED NURSES

With programs proliferating throughout the country, what is the real need for doctorally prepared nurses? Is there sufficient availability of job opportunities for these nurses? Where do they go and what is the demand? Several investigations have studied supply-and-demand issues related to nurses with doctoral degrees. All contend that the need for doctorally prepared nurses will continue to escalate in the future.

The Institute of Medicine (1983) documented a need for doctorally prepared nurses and those with advanced specialization. The Institute identified a serious shortage of nurses with advanced degrees and clinical specialization (p. 149). A concurrent recommendation was to provide federal support and fellowships to enable the growth of the number of nurses with doctoral education.

Anderson, et al. (1985) surveyed baccalaureate and higher-degree programs and documented a substantial demand for doctorally prepared nurses in two areas: (1) academia and (2) health services.

According to their findings, less than 25 percent of nursing faculty in baccalaureate and higher-degree programs in 1983 held an earned doctorate. The authors projected that, in the academic setting alone, the number of nurse doctorates would need to triple in 1988. Cities with large medical centers have a great need for doctorally prepared nurses with expertise in home health, nursing administration, practice, and education. Magnet hospitals were also cited as needing doctorally prepared nurses to work as clinical practitioners.

Perry (1982) emphasized that schools of nursing are a major market for doctorally prepared nurses. She stated that nursing programs must ultimately employ doctorally prepared faculty who are appropriately ready to function as productive scholars in the academic community. She further contended that a person who offers anything less does not qualify for a teaching position. Perry stated:

> I believe that doctoral education creates a qualitative change in the individual experiencing such education. Thus, we are doing a disservice to students who are exposed to instructors without doctoral preparation. (Perry, 1982, p. 96)

Brimmer et al. (1983), in a descriptive, cross-sectional study, reported on education and employment characteristics of nurses with doctoral degrees. Data were obtained in the late 1970s. The authors surveyed participants during three time periods: during doctoral study, in the first position postdoctoral study, and in their current position. Over half of those surveyed (54 percent) earned the PhD degree; 34 percent earned the EdD degree. Education was the major field of study in this population, followed by social/behavioral sciences and nursing. The major institutions awarding degrees "in nursing" were Teachers College, Columbia University (149 degrees), and New York University (103 degrees). Eighty-nine percent of nurses were employed full-time (p. 159). In 1980, baccalaureate programs and higher education employed two-thirds of this population. The remaining nurses were employed, for the most part, in diploma, AD education, in-service, or administrative settings. In reference to current position, most nurses remained in the same type of position, such as baccalaureate or higher-degree education. The largest number worked as teachers (36.4 percent), administrators (33.5 percent), combination teachers/administrators (15.2 percent), clinical work (2.6 percent), and consultation or "other category" (6.9 percent). The mean age of graduates was 41.5 years, and only 6 percent of these individuals were engaged in postdoctoral education. Only 6 percent to 8 percent of doctorally prepared nurses were hired for research. The majority were hired for teaching in baccalaureate and higher-degree programs in nursing. The authors emphasized the need for mentors and appropriate socialization to roles, given the substantial growth in the number of doctorally prepared nurses. Financial support remained critical, including funding for minorities. Demands for higher levels of expertise and the need to build on the group of nurse scholars were cited as crucial.

Amos (1985) noted a need for nurses prepared at the doctoral level to advance the quality of patient care. These nurses can have an impact on the cost of health care. She further stated the need for a core of doctorally prepared nurses in academic health centers.

The need for nurses with doctoral degrees, and where they will make a professional contribution, has been examined. Andreoli (1986) noted that the past decade has produced a demand for doctorally prepared nurses at schools of nursing, academic health centers, community hospitals, and health agencies (p. 66). The National League for Nursing (NLN) (1987) reported that, between 1982 and 1986 alone, the number of students in these programs increased 45 percent. Anderson et al. (1985) reported that a limited number of doctoral programs are available and many qualified applicants cannot be admitted. A tremendous need for nurses with doctorates in academic settings was emphasized.

Career goals will affect nursing supply. Zebelman and Olswang (1989) studied career goal changes of 785 doctoral nursing students in 35 schools in the United States. They surveyed significant differences in career goals between beginning doctoral students and students who had been enrolled in doctoral programs for more than one year. Of primary concern were students whose career goals changed from faculty positions to careers such as research and consultation. The authors found that students in DNS programs were more inclined to be educational administrators, faculty, consultants, and clinical nurse researchers. EdD students were likely to choose careers as educators, administrators, and, especially, faculty in doctoral programs. PhD students were interested in careers as consultants, doctoral faculty, and researchers. Findings indicated that DNS and EdD students do not change their goals from faculty to other types of positions. PhD students do change their goals from faculty to other types of positions (p. 58). Researchers must continue to follow the career goals of doctoral students to determine and predict supply, particularly in faculty positions.

Williams (1989) studied the development of research careers in those seeking a doctorate in nursing. She verbalized great concern about the area of study pursued in doctoral education and the focus of inquiry at the doctoral level. A discrepancy in course of study and research outcomes was noted; the course of study often bore little resemblance to where the individual sought employment. Greater continuity in doctoral study focus and individual career expectations is needed.

Clinical, academic, and community research roles are demands in the nursing marketplace. In academia, a need exists for a supply of nurses with doctorates to educate those interested in both graduate and undergraduate degrees. The quality of patient care will be the ultimate beneficiary of doctoral education, which can have a tremendous impact on health care cost and consumer satisfaction. A strong core of doctorally prepared nurses to develop alternate health care centers is timely in this age of inequitable health care systems.

FUTURE DIRECTIONS FOR RESEARCH

Since the first doctoral program specifically for nurses was developed in the early 1920s at Teachers College, Columbia University, nursing education programs have evolved and diversified in many directions. One of the unanticipated benefits of the doctoral education movement has been a proliferation of programs that seek to strengthen the profession in teaching, research, and practice. The rapid growth of doctoral nursing programs raises concerns about program quality, faculty expertise, and outcomes. The belief that research occurs primarily in PhD nursing programs rather than in other types of doctoral programs is essentially not valid. This was demonstrated in the nursing and non-nursing literature. More similarities than differences in doctoral programs were cited in this literature review. Researchers in both nursing and non-nursing programs should build on this empirical base by designing and conducting investigations that will generate even more substantive data pertaining to outcomes and impact of the varying doctoral programs.

Researchers should take note of the impact doctoral nurses have on practice settings. The impact of these highly educated nurses on the current health care scene could generate federal funding for nurses, to demonstrate how the profession can make a difference in providing equal health care for all people. The critical intervening variables of consumer satisfaction with nurses in advanced clinical practice warrant further investigation.

Questions regarding program quality await continued and further study. Does the profession need accreditation criteria—do quality and excellence issues need further assessment? With the increasing number of doctorally prepared nurses, research efforts should now turn to examining difficult issues such as diversity in doctoral education, which may be the key to richness and quality on this academic level.

REFERENCES

Abdellah, F. (1966). Doctoral preparation for nurses—a continuation of the dialogue. *Nursing Forum, 5,* 33–52.

American Association of Colleges of Nursing's Doctoral Conference. (1985). Consensus for quality. *Journal of Professional Nursing, 1,* 90–100.

American Association of Colleges of Nursing's Doctoral Conference. (1989). A position for nursing in doctoral education: Consensus building. *Journal of Professional Nursing, 5,* 248.

Amos, L. (1985). Issues in doctoral preparation in nursing: Current perspectives and future directions. *Journal of Professional Nursing, 1,* 101–107.

Anderson, C. (1989). Type and expectations of faculty. *Journal of Professional Nursing, 5,* 250–255.

Anderson, E., Roth, P., & Palmer, I. (1985). A national survey of the need for doctorally prepared nurses in academic settings and health service agencies. *Journal of Professional Nursing, 1,* 23–33.

Andreoli, K. (1986). Specialization and graduate curricula: Finding the fit. *Nursing and Health Care, 8,* 65–69.

Barnum, B. J. (1991). Doctoral education for the nurse executive. *Nursing and Health Care Supplement,* Pub. No. 41-2365, 57–59.

Beare, P., Gray, C., & Ptak, H. (1981). Doctoral curricula in nursing. *Nursing Outlook, 29,* 311–316.

Blancett, S. S. (1989). Defining doctoral education. *Nurse Educator, 14,* 3.

Booth, R. (1989). Summary of American Association of Colleges of Nursing's 1989 Doctoral Conference. *Journal of Professional Nursing, 5,* 271–272.

Boston's first doctorate in nursing science goes to nurse midwife. (1963). *American Journal of Nursing, 63,* 8, 27.

Bremner, M., Crutchfield, A., Kosowski, M., Perkins, J., & Williams, G. (1990). Doctoral preparation of nursing faculty. *Nurse Educator, 15,* 12–15.

Brimmer, P., Skoner, M., Pender, N., Williams, C., Fleming, J., & Werley, H. (1983). Nurses with doctoral degrees: Education and employment characteristics. *Research in Nursing and Health, 6,* 157–165.

Brodie, B. (1986). Impact of doctoral programs on nursing education. *Journal of Professional Nursing, 2,* 350–357.

Brown, S. A. (1985). A perspective on why nurses should earn doctorates in nursing. *Perspectives in Psychiatric Care, 1,* 16–21.

Casarett, A. (1989). Components needed to support graduate education. *Journal of Professional Nursing, 5,* 256–260.

Christman, L. (1978). Doctoral education: A shot in the arm for the nursing profession. *Nursing Digest, 6*(2), 45–46.

Cleino, E. (1965). Profile of nurse faculty members with doctoral degrees. *Nursing Outlook, 13,* 37–39.

Cleland, V. (1976). Developing a doctoral program. *Nursing Outlook, 24,* 631–635.

Curran, C., Habeeb, M., & Sobol, E. (1981). Selecting a doctoral program for a career in nursing. *Journal of Nursing Administration, 11,* 35–40.

Downs, F. (1976). Doctoral preparation in nursing: Is it worth it? *Nursing Outlook, 24,* 375–377.

Downs, F. (1978). Doctoral issues in nursing: Future directions. *Nursing Outlook, 26,* 56–61.

Downs, F. (1988). Doctoral education: Our claim to the future. *Nursing Outlook, 36,* 18–20.

Downs, F. (1989). Differences between the professional doctorate and the academic/research doctorate. *Journal of Professional Nursing, 5,* 261–265.

Edens, G. E., & Labadie, G. C. (1987). Opinions about the professional doctorate in nursing. *Nursing Outlook, 35,* 136–140.

Elkins, W. (1960). Doctoral education in nursing—A university president presents his point of view. *Nursing Outlook, 8,* 542–544.

Farren, E. (1991). Doctoral preparation and research productivity. *Nursing Outlook, 39,* 22–25.

Fields, W. (1988). The ultimate nursing doctorate. *Nursing Outlook, 29,* 650–654.

Fitzpatrick, J., Kluznik-Boyle, K., & Anderson, R. (1986). Evaluation of the doctor of nursing (ND) program: Preliminary findings. *Journal of Professional Nursing, 2,* 365–372.

Fitzpatrick, M. L. (1991). Doctoral preparation versus expectations. *Journal of Professional Nursing, 7,* 172–176.

Forni, P. (1989). Models for doctoral programs: First professional degree or terminal degree. *Nursing and Health Care, 10,* 429–434.

Gorney-Fadiman, M. (1981). A student's perspective on the doctoral dilemma. *Nursing Outlook, 29,* 650–654.

Gortner, S. R. (1991). Historical development of doctoral programs: Shaping our expectations. *Journal of Professional Nursing, 7,* 45–53.

Grace, H. K. (1978). The development of doctoral education in nursing: In historical perspective. *Journal of Nursing Education, 17,* 17–27.

Grace, H. K. (1989). Issues in doctoral education in nursing. *Journal of Professional Nursing, 5,* 266–270.

Harris, J., Trout, W., & Andrews, G. (1980). The American doctorate in the context of the new patterns in higher education. Washington, DC: The Council of Postsecondary Accreditation.

Hassenplug, L. (1966). Doctoral preparation for nurses—A continuation of the dialogue. *Nursing Forum, 5,* 53–56.

Holzemer, B. (1987). Doctoral education in nursing: An assessment of quality, 1979–1984. *Nursing Research, 36,* 111–116.

Holzemer, W., & Chambers, D. (1986). Healthy nursing doctoral programs: Relationship between perceptions of the academic environment and productivity of faculty and alumni. *Research in Nursing and Health, 9,* 299–307.

Institute of Medicine. (1983). Nursing and nursing education: Public policies and private actions. Washington: National Academy Press.

Kemble, E. (1966). Doctoral preparation for nurses: A continuation of the dialogue. *Nursing Forum, 5,* 39–44.

Ketefian, S. (1991). Doctoral preparation for faculty roles: Expectations and realities. *Journal of Professional Nursing, 7,* 105–111.

Lash, A. (1987a). The nature of the doctor of philosophy degree: Evolving conceptions. *Journal of Professional Nursing, 3,* 92–101.

Lash, A. (1987b). Rival conceptions in doctoral education in nursing and their outcomes: An update. *Journal of Nursing Education, 26,* 221–227.

Leininger, M. (1976). Doctoral programs for nurses: Trends, questions, and projected plans. *Nursing Research, 25,* 201–210.

Loomis, M. (1985). Emerging content in nursing—an analysis of dissertation abstracts and titles, 1976–1982. *Nursing Research, 34,* 113–116.

Lutz, E., & Schlotfeldt, R. (1985). Pioneering a new approach to professional education. *Nursing Outlook, 33,* 139–143.

Marriner-Tomey, A. (1990). Historical development of doctoral programs from the Middle Ages to nursing education today. *Nursing and Health Care, 11,* 133–137.

Matarazzo, J., & Abdellah, F. (1971). Doctoral education for nurses in the United States. *Nursing Research, 20,* 404–414.

McManus, L. (1960). Doctoral education in nursing—a nurse educator responds. *Nursing Outlook, 8*(10), 543–545.

Meleis, A. (1988). Doctoral education in nursing: Its present and future. *Journal of Professional Nursing, 4,* 436–446.

Moccia, P. (1986). DSN debate. *Nursing and Health Care,* 265.

Murphy, J. (1981). Doctoral education in, of, and for nursing: An historical analysis. *Nursing Outlook, 29,* 645–648.

Murphy, J. (1984). Essential resources for developing doctoral programs in nursing, *Nurse Educator,* 7–10.

Murphy, J. (1985). Doctoral education of nurses: Historical developments, programs and graduates. *Research in Nursing Education,* 171–188.

Nahm, H. (1966). Doctoral preparation for nurses—a continuation of the dialogue. *Nursing Forum, 5,* 37–39.

National League for Nursing. (1987). *Nursing data review.* New York: NLN.

Newman, M. (1975). The professional doctorate in nursing: Position paper. *Nursing Outlook, 23,* 704–706.

Norris, C. (1985). The PhD in nursing program: A five-year projection . . . faculty in those schools. *Nurse Educator, 10* (2), 6–11.

Parietti, E. S. (1979). *Development of doctoral education for nurses: An historical survey.* Unpublished doctoral dissertation, Teachers College, Columbia University.

Peplau, H. (1966). Nursing's two routes to doctoral degrees. *Nursing Forum, 5,* 51–67.

Perry, S. (1982, February). A doctorate—necessary but not sufficient. *Nursing Outlook,* 95–98.

Pitel, M., & Vian, J. (1975). Analysis of nurse doctorates. *Nursing Research, 24,* 340–351.

Position statement—indicators of quality in doctor programs in nursing. (1987). *Journal of Professional Nursing,* 72–74.

Robertson, N. L., & Sistler, J. K. (1971). *The doctorate in education.* Bloomington, IN: Phi Delta Kappa and the American Association of Colleges for Teacher Education.

Rogers, M. (1966). Doctoral education in nursing. *Nursing Forum, 5,* 75–82.

Schlotfeldt, R. (1966). Doctoral study in basic disciplines. *Nursing Forum, 5,* 68–74.

Schlotfeldt, R. (1978). The professional doctorate: Rationale and characteristics. *Nursing Outlook, 26,* 302–311.

Seitz, P. (1987, May). The pros and cons of doctoral education. *The Canadian Nurse,* 27.

Shores, L. (1986). Analysis of decisions to initiate doctoral programs in nursing. *Nurse Educator, 11,* 26–30.

Snyder-Halpern, R. (1986). Nursing doctorates: Is there a difference? *Nursing Outlook, 34,* 284–286.

Taylor, S., Gifford, A., & Vian, J. (1971). Nurses with earned doctoral degrees. *Nursing Research, 20*(5), 415–427.

VanDongen, C. J. (1988). The life experience of the first year doctoral student. *Nurse Educator, 13,* 19–23.

Werley, H., & Leske, J. (1988). Pinning down the tracks to doctoral degrees. *Nursing and Health Care, 9,* 239–243.

Wiley, K. (1989). Focus of research for PhD in nursing. *Journal of Nursing Education, 28,* 190–192.

Williams, C. (1989). Doctoral programs in nursing and the development of research careers. *Journal of Professional Nursing, 5,* 117–168.

Zebelman, E. S., & Olswang, S. G. (1989). Student career goal changes during doctoral education in nursing. *Journal of Nursing Education, 28,* 53–59.

Zeimer, M., Brown, J., Fitzpatrick, M. L., Manfredi, C., O'Leary, J., & Valiga, T. (1992). Doctoral programs in nursing: Philosophy, curricula, and program requirements. *Journal of Professional Nursing, 8,* (1), 56–62.

Chapter Four

EMPATHY: THEORY, RESEARCH, AND NURSING APPLICATIONS

Janice M. Layton, PhD, RN

INTRODUCTION

Over the past several decades, beginning with the work of Carl Rogers and his associates, a theory of empathy has gradually evolved (Rogers, 1957; Rogers, Gendlin, Kiesler, & Truax, 1967; Truax & Carkhuff, 1967). Initially, Rogers (1957) identified empathy, warmth, and genuineness as the three qualities required of a therapist to provide the necessary and sufficient conditions for therapeutic growth to occur. In a later article, Rogers (1975, p. 3) noted that "over the years . . . the research evidence . . . points strongly to the conclusion that a high degree of empathy in a relationship is possibly *the* most potent and certainly one of the most potent factors in bringing about change and learning."

Recent theories have focused on empathy as a process consisting of steps or stages. Several nurse researchers have entered into this discussion with parallel or similar models. Kunst-Wilson, Carpenter, Poser, Venohr, and Kushner (1981) portrayed empathy as consisting of two stages: (1) perception and (2) action. The perceptual component centers on detecting and identifying the feelings of the client. The action component entails using the information to benefit the client. LaMonica (1981) also proposed a stage or process theory of empathy. "The helper must first perceive, then communicate perceptions to the client, and then the client must perceive understanding from the helper" (p. 399). Reynolds and Presly (1988) used the terms trait empathy and state or interactional empathy. Trait empathy and state empathy are similar to but not the same as stages of empathy. Recent nursing theories mirror earlier nursing theorists such as Zderad (1969) and Ehmann (1971), both of whom distinguished natural or raw empathy from its clinical application.

Alligood (1991) and Wheeler (1988) incorporated the concept of empathy into their application of Martha Rogers' science of unitary human beings. Alligood (1991) viewed empathy as related to or derived from the principle of integrality, that is, as a human field pattern characterizing human–environment interaction. She measured empathy using Hogan's (1969) empathy scale, which was designed to measure empathy as a trait or characteristic of a person. Thus, Alligood operationally defined empathy as a trait. This view is consistent with the stage theories of empathy and also with those theories that divide empathy into a trait and a state. In a later article, Alligood (1992) stressed the importance of distinguishing trait or basic empathy from the clinical or trained state of empathy.

THE PROCESS OF EMPATHY

Empathy as a process occurring in stages has been most clearly delineated by Barrett-Lennard (1981). He viewed empathy as occurring in the following sequence of phases: (1) empathic resonation (active attending and listening with an empathic set), (2) expressed empathy, and (3) received empathy. Empathic set is a precondition for Phase 1 and might also be thought of as natural or trait empathy. Barrett-Lennard included a postcondition of feedback to the helper, which brings the empathic interaction back to Phase 1.

Gladstein (1983, 1987) expanded theoretical explorations of empathy beyond the counseling literature to the fields of developmental and social psychology. He found that each of these three fields has its own body of literature and instruments and that there is little overlap among the fields. He noted, though, that each of the three specialties has the same two models of empathy: (1) role taking and (2) emotional contagion. Role taking is a cognitive process of intellectually putting oneself in another's place; it might be included as part of empathic set and Phase 1 in the Barrett-Lennard model. Emotional contagion is affective empathy and is an emotional response that may lead to expressed empathy (Phase 2 in the Barrett-Lennard model). Role taking and emotional contagion do not fit neatly into Barrett-Lennard's phases. They are more like parallel processes underlying paths to empathy: one can connect with others either intellectually or emotionally or in both ways. Rogers' original ideas of empathy included both intellectual and emotional components.

Gladstein also pointed out that a very strong affective response may result in the helper's wanting to distance himself or herself. This observation of Gladstein underscores the complexity of the empathic process and the fact that empathy does not always lead to helping behavior. Katz (1963) outlined barriers or reasons why helpers may not demonstrate empathy. The first barrier is anxiety, such as that produced by unmet needs and unresolved personal conflicts. In its extreme form, anxiety over dealing constantly with serious and demanding situations can result in the protective mechanism of burnout. Tyner (1985) and Williams (1989) referred to such a process. A second barrier is an authoritarian attitude, that is, being in a position of power and control. This is a serious pitfall for clinicians, whose position assumes they are authorities. The third barrier is trying too hard to be professional, which may lead to focusing on technique rather than on the patient. The fourth barrier is problems in a particular situation, such as personality clashes or differences related to social class, culture, or age. Gould (1990) suggested that these barriers, as outlined by Katz, prevented empathy from being expressed by nurses.

In a similar vein, Gallop, Lancee, and Garfinkel (1990) suggested mediating variables underlying the early phases of empathy. Using Barrett-Lennard's (1981) model as a framework, they discussed variables that may occur through the phase of expressing empathy that result in different outcomes, such as terminating an interaction or demonstrating understanding.

Recent nurse authors and theorists have questioned the appropriateness of empathy in nursing practice. Pike (1990) suggested that the concept of caring replaces the concept of empathy. Diers (1990), however, pointed out that nurses draw on a wide range of knowledge and skills and cautioned against replacing empathy as a broad concept with caring as a broad concept.

Morse et al. (1992) and Morse, Bottorff, Anderson, O'Brien, and Solberg (1992), in their comprehensive and thoughtful analyses, presented a model that includes both cognitive and emotional empathy but is much broader; it extends to other responses and behaviors as well. Their model included the spontaneous, emotional responses of the nurse, such as pity and sympathy, as well as learned responses, such as therapeutic empathy and humor. Also included were self-focused responses, both natural (withdrawing and dehumanizing) and learned (false reassurance and rote behavior). They pointed out that therapeutic empathy may not be appropriate or needed by patients, especially in acute care settings, and that other responses may be more helpful.

Table 1 represents the relationship among some of the empathy frameworks and theories and compares them to Barrett-Lennard (1981), which is the most comprehensive theory. Readers should note that, although Gladstein (1983, 1987) is included, his theory does not fit as well as the others, all of which are stage theories.

Table 1. Relationship of Selected Empathy Frameworks to Barrett-Lennard's Phase Theory

		Phase 1	Phase 2	Phase 3
Barrett-Lennard (1981)	Empathic Set	Empathic Resonance	Expressed Empathy	Received Feedback Empathy
Kunst-Wilson, Carpenter, Poser, Venohr, & Kushner (1981)		Perception	Action	
LaMonica (1981)		Helper Perception	Helper Communication	Client Perception
Reynolds & Presley (1988)	Trait	State or Interactional		
Ehmann (1971)	Raw	Clinical ———	———	———
Zderad (1969)	Natural	Clinical ———	———	———
Gladstein (1983; 1987)	——— ———	Role Taking (Cognitive) ——— Emotional Contagion (Affective) ———	——— ———	——— ———

THE MEASUREMENT OF EMPATHY

The refinement of theories of empathy has advanced research on empathy, especially its measurement, which is the most difficult aspect of empathy research. Historically, the measurement of empathy has been a picture of confusion with a number of tests available, intercorrelations of which were low to moderate. Barrett-Lennard's (1981) division of empathy into phases provided a way to organize the potpourri of empathy tests that are used in different studies, as well as a rationale for selecting appropriate instruments.

Barrett-Lennard (1981) asserted that different phases of empathy should be measured differently. He noted that there are no well-established measures of Phase 1, empathic set and active attending. He suggested that the most commonly used measure of Phase 2, expressed empathy, is the Carkhuff (1969a, 1969b) scale, as used by independent judges. He recommended the client form of the Barrett-Lennard (1962) Relationship Inventory (BLRI) for Phase 3, received empathy. LaMonica's (1981) Empathy Construct Rating Scale (ECRS), which is similar in format to the BLRI, was also developed as a measure of received empathy for use specifically in patient care settings. The LaMonica (1986) Empathy Profile (LEP), a derivative of the ECRS, is a forced-choice, self-report instrument with five subscales representing different helping modes.

Although Barrett-Lennard (1981) felt there were no well-established measures of Phase 1, others have used the Hogan (1969) Empathy Scale (Alligood, 1991; Reynolds & Presly, 1988) or the Kagan Affective Sensitivity Scale (Schneider, Hastorf, & Ellsworth, 1979). Layton and Wykle (1990) also suggested the Empathy Test might be a measure of Phase 1. The Empathy Test taps knowledge of principles of empathy and would be appropriate if empathic set was broadened to include cognitive variables. Self-ratings on the BLRI and the ECRS are also used as Phase 1 measures. Table 2 summarizes the instruments that are suggested to measure each phase of empathy.

Construct Validity

A key issue in research involving empathy is the construct validity of the tests used to measure the empathy variable. Various methods have been developed to assess construct validity. The major approaches, according to Messick (1989), are correlational and multitrait–multimethod analyses and factor analytic and group difference studies.

Table 2. Instruments Measuring Differnt Phases of Empathy

Phase 1	Phase 2	Phase 3
BLRI—self-rating	Carkhuff scale	BLRI—client rating
ECRS—self-rating		ECRS—client rating
Hogan		
Kagan Affective Sensitivity Scale		
Empathy Test		

Note: Phase 1 includes empathic set.

The results of correlational studies of empathy measures are mixed. Kurtz and Grummon (1972), correlating scores from six empathy instruments, found a moderate relationship during therapy between the empathy subtest of the BLRI (client-perceived) and tape-judged empathy using the Carkhuff scale ($r = .31$, $p < .10$, $N = 31$). However, near the end of therapy, the correlation was zero. Layton (1979) found moderate correlations between scores on the same two instruments at two points in time ($r = .27$ and $r = .31$, $p < .05$, $N = 56$). Subsequently, Layton and Wykle (1990), evaluating the construct validity of four empathy instruments, found the Carkhuff scale significantly correlated with the ECRS ($r = .37$, $p < .01$, $N = 50$) and the Empathy Test ($r = .25$, $p < .05$). The ECRS and BLRI were also significantly correlated ($r = .78$, $p < .001$). (The latter correlation is inflated from similarity of method.) Jarski, Gjerde, Bratton, Brown, and Matthes (1985) found correlations between scores on Hornblow's general empathy rating, the Carkhuff scale, and the BLRI ($r = .60–.76$, $p < .001$, $N = 60$). As discussed below, the correlations in various studies, which range from low to high, are consistent with the phase theories of empathy.

A number of studies have examined group differences on empathy measures. Stetler (1977), whose study included diploma, associate degree, and baccalaureate-prepared nurses, found no relationship between empathy and age or educational background of registered nurses. Forsyth (1979), however, found that level of education and empathy were positively correlated, with baccalaureate-prepared nurses demonstrating higher levels of empathy than diploma or associate degree nurses. Kunst-Wilson et al. (1981), comparing different educational levels from freshman baccalaureate through graduate nursing students, found that educational level was a significant predictor of empathic ability. Layton (1979) and Layton and Wykle (1990) found that senior baccalaureate nursing students were more empathic than junior students and that registered nurses scored significantly higher than nursing assistants on different empathy measures.

The results of the various studies on tests measuring empathy fit well with the phase theories of empathy discussed earlier. Most studies revealed modest correlations between measures of Phase 1 and Phase 2 empathy and also between Phase 2 and Phase 3. High correlations were noted in one study (Layton & Wykle, 1990) between two Phase 3 measures, the BLRI and the ECRS. Low correlations were found between Phase 1 and Phase 3 measures. The low correlations between Phases 1 and 3 and the higher correlations between Phases 1 and 2 and Phases 2 and 3 are not surprising. They are, rather, an expectation consistent with the theory that empathy occurs in stages. The tests are measuring related but slightly different variables, and the closer the variables or phases, the higher the correlations.

EMPATHY IN NURSING

Studies in the area of empathy in nursing and nursing education are of relatively recent origin. For the past 20 to 25 years, a small body of empathy research by and about nurses has been accumulating. LaMonica (1979) pointed out the necessity for empathy in the nurse–client relationship. Following Rogers' and Carkhuff's line of thinking, she delineated two phases in a helping relationship: (1) understanding the client and building the relationship, and (2) using the relationship to help the client change. LaMonica (1979) emphasized that "empathy is the primary condition in the comprehensive helping process and operates in every facet of an interaction" (p. 4). Finding existing empathy measures inadequate for patient care settings, LaMonica (1981) developed the ECRS.

In a landmark field experiment, LaMonica, Wolf, Madea, and Oberst (1987) evaluated the effects of nurse empathy instruction on selected patient outcomes with cancer patients and the results of instruction on the empathy level of the nurses. The dependent variables of anxiety, hostility, depression, and satisfaction with care were measured before and after the empathy instruction and the control instruction given to the nurses. Nurses' empathy was also measured before and after instruction; a four-group design was used to control for pretest effects. The patient subjects showed significant decreases in anxiety and hostility and nonsignificant differences in the predicted direction for depression and satisfaction with care. The changes in the patients, attributed to the empathy instruction the nurses received, were judged to have considerable clinical significance because the patients were all under treatment for cancer.

One unexpected finding in the LaMonica et al. (1987) study was that the empathy instruction did not produce an increase in empathy scores in the nurse subjects. Scores on the ECRS in all subjects were high both before and after training, suggesting a ceiling effect. Rawnsley (1987), in her response to the reported research, had some interesting observations on the high empathy scores. (Her observations are pertinent to comments made earlier in this chapter, regarding types and phases of empathy.) She suggested that the nurses had a high degree of natural empathy prior to training and that possibly the clinical environment helped foster empathy. Rawnsley cautioned against viewing empathy only as a quantitative construct and advised continued development of empathy from a theoretical point of view.

In another field study, Reid-Ponte (1992) examined the relationship of nurses' empathy to cancer patients' distress. Empathy was measured using LaMonica's (1986) Empathy Profile (LEP). The hypothesis that empathy would be negatively related to distress was supported. Both empathy and distress levels were low, however, and, on some of the LEP subscales, the direction of the correlation was positive rather than negative. The author pointed out that patients' distress may increase as nurses convey empathy.

Several studies have examined empathy with gerontological clients in different settings. Bagshaw and Adams (1986) investigated the relationships among three variables: (1) empathy, as measured by the ECRS, (2) attitudes toward older people, and (3) custodial vs. therapeutic orientation toward treatment. Subjects were registered nurses (RNs), licensed practical nurses (LPNs), and nursing assistants (NAs). The investigators found correlations among low empathy, negative attitudes toward older people, and a custodial attitude toward treatment. Positive attitudes toward older people were not correlated with high empathy, however. RNs were more empathic and less custodial and negative in attitudes than LPNs or NAs. LPNs scored better than NAs. There were also significant differences among the seven nursing homes sampled, indicating an environmental or context effect.

Pennington and Pierce (1985) studied whether selected demographic variables could predict empathy in employees of long-term care facilities for the elderly. During interactions with residents, staff were judged by trained raters using the Carkhuff scale. A moderate amount (1 to 5 years) of work experience was the only significant predictor of empathy. The correlation of empathy and age approached significance ($p < .053$), with younger persons being more empathic. The authors suggested that burnout may explain why long-time employees demonstrated little empathy.

Schirm and Fennell (1991) examined the empathy of home health nurses caring for elderly clients and the relationship of this empathy to the strain of the family caregivers. They found that home health nurses rated with the ECRS were highly empathic, although the correlation between empathy and family caregiver strain was not significant. Nurses in rural settings were rated higher on empathy than those in suburban settings. Possibly, rural families relied more on the nurses.

Dawson (1985) predicted that hypertensive patients would perceive less empathy, compared with diabetics or a control group, and that they would have more difficulty with self-disclosure. Hypertensives did perceive less empathy, as measured by the BLRI, than the other groups, but did not differ on self-disclosure. The author commented that failure to perceive empathy has serious treatment implications, because hypertensives tend to develop private "theories" about whether treatment is effective.

In two studies, the difference in empathy of nurses working in different settings was examined. Sparling and Jones (1977) noted that nurses working in a psychiatric setting were more empathic than nurses working in a medical-surgical setting, and that educational level, age, experience, gender, and marital status did not make a difference in empathy. Brunt (1985) discovered, contrary to his prediction, that nurses working in intensive care settings did not have lower empathy than nurses working in nonintensive care settings. He did find that number of years working on a unit was negatively related to empathy. Two observations are offered regarding the relationship of setting to empathy:

1. Stage theories do not take environment into account. The history of behaviorism, however, teaches that environment is a powerful determinant of behavior.
2. The negative correlation of empathy to number of years in a setting is consistent with the research on empathy and burnout

discussed under barriers to empathy and elsewhere. Researchers should at least be aware of the influence of these contextual variables in empathy studies.

LaMonica, Carew, Winder, Haase, and Blanchard (1976) tested an empathy education program on nurse subjects who scored low in empathy. The educational program was effective in increasing the nurses' ability to perceive and to respond with empathy. Even though the increase was statistically significant, however, most subjects remained below what was considered a minimal therapeutic level of empathy. Elsewhere, LaMonica and Karshmer (1978) demonstrated that senior baccalaureate nursing students also scored low on empathy and that their course in psychiatric nursing raised them to therapeutic levels. The authors recommended that empathy be taught in educational and health care settings. LaMonica and Karshmer (1978) and LaMonica (1983) outlined an educational program to increase empathy levels. The program, based on the human relations training model, incorporates didactic instruction, experiential learning, modeling, rehearsal, feedback, and imagery.

Hill and Knowles (1983), using the Carkhuff scale, likewise found nurses low in empathy, but noted higher scores among those who had had supervised practice in interpersonal relations.

Layton (1979) used Bandura's theory of modeling to teach empathy to nursing students. Based on the notion that most complex behavior is learned by observing others, Layton tested various modeling conditions and found that covert rehearsal or mental practice significantly improved empathy. Hodges (1991) found no effect from empathy instruction that incorporated role modeling, role playing, and didactic and experiential learning.

Relating education to a division of empathy into trait and state or interactional empathy, Reynolds (1987), after reviewing a number of studies, concluded that state or interactional empathy might be increased by instruction, but that trait empathy is not easily changed. Reynolds noted that state empathy (measured by the ECRS) but not trait empathy (measured by the Hogan scale) changed during a three-month educational program in two or three colleges of nursing.

Rogers (1986) surveyed sophomore, junior, and senior baccalaureate students in two nursing programs. There were nonsignificant improvements in empathy (with the exception of one class in one school) as students progressed through the program. Students' self-ratings and ratings by patients, all measured using the ECRS, revealed generally high empathy scores, indicating a possible ceiling effect.

Kirk and Thomas (1982) instructed psychiatric nurses using Interpersonal Process Recall. The experimental group, compared to a no-treatment control, performed better on the Kagan Affective Sensitivity Scale and self and patient ratings using the BLRI. No differences were found on supervisor ratings using the Carkhuff scale. The researchers considered the differences detected by patients to be especially significant.

CONCLUSIONS AND RECOMMENDATIONS

Several suggestions are offered for all studies of empathy. Research involving empathy should always be carried out within a theoretical framework, to enhance development and testing of the theories. Use of theory also offers other advantages: research designed within a theoretical context is more meaningful, and comparisons across studies are facilitated. A specific theory is not recommended: researchers should choose one that seems most suited to their particular background and interests.

Closely related to use of theory is careful attention to measurement. Instruments selected should fit with the theory. For example, if a stage theory is used, tests must be consistent with the stage being measured. Or, if empathy as a trait is being studied, a trait measure is indicated. Construct validation studies are needed, but a validation component can be incorporated into many studies with little additional effort. For example, if two empathy instruments are used, correlation of scores on the two tests can be done and the results can be interpreted within the theoretical framework of the study.

Given the problems of measuring psychosocial variables, including empathy, researchers are advised to be aware of the psychometric properties of the empathy instruments. Reliability should be checked with every use, because it can vary from group to group. Scores clustering at the high or low end of the scale should be addressed. Ceiling effects have been noted in several studies, and it is not clear whether this effect is a property of the instrument or reflects true high scores of the participants. Patients' ratings of nurses sometimes yield very high scores, calling these ratings into question. Use of simulated patients is one way to obtain more objective measurement until better approaches are developed to seek input from actual patients.

As to the method and design of empathy research, many approaches are needed. Quantitative studies continue to be required, and the newer qualitative approaches are yielding rich data and intuitively appealing theories. It is not a question of either–or: quantitative and qualitative approaches supplement each other and, if used together, will eventually lead to better theoretical understanding of empathy in nursing. Quantitative methods have a longer history in nursing, but qualitative approaches are needed to accurately depict the complexity of nursing, especially in the interpersonal realm.

Some of the nursing problems to be addressed are suggested by the studies reviewed in this paper. Outcome studies, or the effects of empathy with particular groups of patients, are needed. Satisfaction with care and adherence to treatment are two of the many possible outcomes that might be studied. Patients with chronic problems, such as cancer, AIDS, hypertension, and heart disease, who are in great need of empathic nursing care, have been included in some studies. However, anyone with a health care crisis needs good nursing, including empathy and other interpersonal skills. Patients might also be selected on the basis of specific nursing problems or diagnoses rather than medical diagnoses. As nursing systems become better developed and more standardized, selection of patients using a nursing framework will be possible.

Context or environmental effects and the interaction of environmental and intrapsychic factors are other topics for future study. The relationship of empathy to particular care settings is a vast area, given the ever-increasing types of settings in which nurses work. The effect of burnout on nurses' empathy is one environmental variable on which research has begun.

Finally, ways to increase nurses' empathy should continue to be examined. Various instructional approaches are discussed in the studies reviewed here. Empathy research in nursing began with educational studies; today, more clinical studies are being carried out. Both continue to be needed as empathy and the interpersonal aspect of nursing are recognized for their critical role in patient care.

REFERENCES

Alligood, M. (1991). Testing Rogers' theory of accelerating change: The relationship among creativity, actualization, and empathy in persons 18–92 years of age. *Western Journal of Nursing Research, 13*, 84–96.

Alligood, M. (1992). Empathy: The importance of recognizing two types. *Journal of Psychosocial Nursing, 30,* 14–17.

Bagshaw, M., & Adams, M. (1986). Nursing home nurses' attitudes, empathy, and ideologic orientation. *International Journal of Aging and Human Development, 22,* 235–246.

Barrett-Lennard, G. T. (1962). Dimensions of therapist response as causal factors in the therapeutic change. *Psychological Monographs, 76,* 43. (Whole No. 562.)

Barrett-Lennard, G. T. (1981). The empathy cycle: Refinement of a nuclear concept. *Journal of Counseling Psychology, 28,* 91–100.

Brunt, J. H. (1985). An exploration of the relationship between nurses' empathy and technology. *Nursing Administration Quarterly, 9,* 69–78.

Carkhuff, R. (1969a). *Helping and human relations: Vol. 1. Selection and training.* New York: Holt, Rinehart and Winston.

Carkhuff, R. (1969b). *Helping and human relations: Vol. 2. Practice and research.* New York: Holt, Rinehart and Winston.

Dawson, C. (1985). Hypertension, perceived clinician empathy, and patient self-disclosure. *Research in Nursing & Health, 8,* 191–198.

Diers, D. (1990). Response. *Journal of Professional Nursing, 6,* 240–241.

Ehmann, V. E. (1971). Empathy: Its origin, characteristics, and process. *Perspectives in Psychiatric Care, 9,* 72–80.

Forsyth, G. L. (1979). Exploration of empathy in nurse–client interaction. *Advances in Nursing Science, 1,* 53–61.

Gallop, R., Lancee, W. J., & Garfinkel, P. E. (1990). The empathic process and its mediators: A heuristic model. *The Journal of Nervous and Mental Diseases, 178,* 649–654.

Gladstein, G. A. (1983). Understanding empathy: Integrating counseling, developmental, and social psychology perspectives, *Journal of Counseling Psychology, 30,* 467–482.

Gladstein, G. A. (1987). The role of empathy in counseling: Theoretical considerations. In G. A. Gladstein and Associates, *Empathy and counseling: Exploration in theory and research* (pp. 1–20). New York: Springer-Verlag.

Gould, D. (1990). Empathy: A review of the literature with suggestions for an alternative research strategy. *Journal of Advanced Nursing, 15,* 1167–1174.

Hill, M. D., & Knowles, D. (1983). Nurses' level of empathy and respect in simulated interactions with patients. *International Journal of Nursing Studies, 20,* 83–87.

Hodges, S. A. (1991). An experiment in the development of empathy in student nurses. *Journal of Advanced Nursing, 16,* 1296–1300.

Hogan, R. (1969). Development of an empathy scale. *Journal of Counseling and Clinical Psychology, 33,* 307–315.

Jarski, R. W., Gjerde, C. L., Bratton, D. B., Brown, D. D., & Matthes, S. S. (1985). A comparison of four empathy instruments in simulated patient–medical student interactions. *Journal of Medical Education, 60,* 545–552.

Katz, R. L. (1963). *Empathy: Its nature and uses.* London: Free Press/ Macmillan.

Kirk, W. G., & Thomas, A. H. (1982). A brief in-service training strategy to increase levels of empathy of psychiatric nursing personnel. *Journal of Psychiatric Treatment and Evaluation, 4,* 177–179.

Kunst-Wilson, W., Carpenter, L., Poser, A., Venohr, I., & Kushner, K. (1981). Empathic perceptions of nursing students: Self-reported and actual ability. *Research in Nursing & Health, 4,* 283–293.

Kurtz, R. R., & Grummon, D. L. (1972). Different approaches to the measurement of therapist empathy and their relationship to therapy outcomes. *Journal of Consulting and Clinical Psychology, 39,* 106–115.

LaMonica, E. L. (1979). Empathy in nursing practice. *Issues in Mental Health Nursing, 2,* 1–13.

LaMonica, E. L. (1981). Construct validity of an empathy instrument. *Research in Nursing & Health, 4,* 389–400.

LaMonica, E. L. (1983). Empathy can be learned. *Nurse Educator, 8*(2), 19–23.

LaMonica, E. L. (1986). *The LaMonica Empathy Profile.* Tuxedo, NY: Xicom.

LaMonica, E. L., Carew, D. K., Winder, A. E., Haase, A. M., & Blanchard, K. H. (1976). Empathy training as the major thrust of a staff development program. *Nursing Research, 25,* 447–451.

LaMonica, E. L., & Karshmer, J. F. (1978). Empathy: Educating nurses in professional practice. *Journal of Nursing Education, 17,* 3–11.

LaMonica, E. L., Wolf, R. M., Madea, A. R., & Oberst, M. T. (1987). Empathy and nursing care outcomes. *Scholarly Inquiry for Nursing Practice: An International Journal, 1,* 197–213.

Layton, J. M. (1979). The use of modeling to teach empathy to nursing students. *Research in Nursing & Health, 2,* 163–176.

Layton, J. M., & Wykle, M. H. (1990). A validity study of four empathy instruments. *Research in Nursing & Health, 13,* 319–325.

Messick, S. (1989). Validity. In R. L. Linn (Ed.), *Educational measurement* (3rd ed.) (pp. 13–103). New York: American Council on Education/Macmillan.

Morse, J. M., Anderson, G., Bottorff, J., Yonge, O., O'Brien, B., Solberg, S. M., & McIlveen, K. H. (1992). Exploring empathy: A conceptual fit for nursing practice? *Image: The Journal of Nursing Scholarship, 24,* 273–280.

Morse, J. M., Bottorff, J., Anderson, G., O'Brien, B., & Solberg, S. (1992). Beyond empathy: Expanding expressions of caring. *Journal of Advanced Nursing, 17,* 809–821.

Pennington, R. E., & Pierce, W. L. (1985). Observations of empathy of nursing-home staff: A predictive study. *International Journal of Aging and Human Development, 2,* 281–290.

Pike, A. W. (1990). On the nature and place of empathy in clinical nursing practice. *Journal of Professional Nursing, 6,* 235–240.

Rawnsley, M. M. (1987). Response to "Empathy and Nursing Care Outcomes." *Scholarly Inquiry for Nursing Practice: An International Journal, 1,* 215–219.

Reid-Ponte, P. (1992). Distress in cancer patients and primary nurses' empathy skills. *Cancer Nursing, 15,* 283–292.

Reynolds, W. J. (1987). Empathy: We know what we mean, but what do we teach? *Nurse Education Today, 7,* 265–269.

Reynolds, W. J., & Presly, A. S. (1988). A study of empathy in student nurses. *Nurse Education Today, 8,* 123–130.

Rogers, C. R. (1957). The necessary and sufficient conditions for therapeutic change. *Journal of Consulting Psychology, 21,* 95–103.

Rogers, C. R. (1975). Empathic: An unappreciated way of being. *Counseling Psychologist, 5,* 2–10.

Rogers, C. R., Gendlin, E., Kiesler, D., & Truax, C. B. (Eds.). (1967). *The therapeutic relationship and its impact.* Madison: University of Wisconsin Press.

Rogers, I. A. (1986). The effect of undergraduate nursing education on empathy. *Western Journal of Nursing Research, 8,* 329–342.

Schirm, V., & Fennell, S. (1991). Nurse empathy to caregivers of chronically ill elders. *Journal of Gerontological Nursing, 17,* 18–22.

Schneider, D., Hastorf, A., & Ellsworth, P. (1979). *Person perception.* Reading, MA: Addison-Wesley.

Sparling, S. L., & Jones, S. L. (1977). Setting: A contextual variable associated with empathy. *Journal of Psychiatric Nursing and Mental Health Services, 15*(4), 9–12.

Stetler, C. B. (1977). Relationships of perceived empathy to nurses' communication. *Nursing Research, 26,* 432–438.

Truax, C. B., & Carkhuff, R. (1967). *Toward effective counseling and psychotherapy.* Chicago: Aldine.

Tyner, R. (1985). Elements of empathic care for dying patients and their families. *Nursing Clinics of North America, 20*(2), 393–401.

Wheeler, K. (1988). A nursing science approach to understanding empathy. *Archives of Psychiatric Nursing, 2,* 95–102.

Williams, C. A. (1989). Empathy and burnout in male and female helping professionals. *Research in Nursing & Health, 12,* 169–178.

Zderad, L. T. (1969). Empathic nursing: Realization of human capacity. *Nursing Clinics of North America, 4*(4), 655–662.

Chapter Five

RETENTION OF NURSING STUDENTS: INTERVENTION STRATEGIES

Bonnie L. Saucier, PhD, RN

INTRODUCTION

Because a continuing shortage of nurses, fluctuations in nursing school enrollments, and an increase in the numbers of underrepresented populations, the retention of nursing students has been of primary concern to schools of nursing for several years. Attrition rates and factors relating to enrollments further emphasize the need for innovative and effective retention programs, if educators wish to assist in alleviating the nursing shortage through increased numbers of graduates. Heydman (1991) summarized findings in the literature regarding the problems and issues of attrition and retention. The literature was critiqued to provide direction for future research. It was concluded that the nursing research literature provided limited direction for nurse educators to improve retention of students. In this chapter, specific retention strategy studies will be reviewed.

A review of the literature suggests that several themes regarding retention have developed since 1990. Several studies address strategies indicated for successful retention of nursing students. National statistics are available to confirm enrollments and further direct trends for retention strategies, particularly among underrepresented populations (National League for Nursing, 1991).

Over a five-year period, in general, associate degree programs have demonstrated increased enrollments; baccalaureate enrollments have decreased since 1988. There has been a steady increase of master's student enrollments and doctoral student enrollments and graduations. Continuous analysis of enrollments and graduations is necessary in order to predict recruitment and retention figures.

In 1989's Fall term, there were increases in enrollments in all three types of undergraduate nursing programs. Associate degree programs led the growth with a 10.6 percent rise from 1988. Diploma programs reported an increase of 8.3 percent in enrollments over 1988. Enrollments in basic baccalaureate programs rose 6.8 percent (National League for Nursing, 1991).

The American Association of Colleges of Nursing (1992) reported changes in enrollment for both 1990 and 1991. Baccalaureate program enrollments decreased by 7.0 percent, and enrollment in master's, generic master's, and doctoral programs increased. Graduations from master's programs increased slightly (4.8 percent). There was a dramatic increase in generic master's graduations (44.2 percent). Doctoral student graduations increased by 21 percent.

Regional distribution of graduates from basic nursing programs in 1989 indicated that the South produced approximately one-third of the nation's new nurses; another 28 percent originated from the Midwest, 24 percent came from the Northeast, and 16 percent from the West (National League for Nursing, 1991). An American Association of Colleges of Nursing (1992) report further indicated that there were enrollment changes by region: baccalaureate program enrollments decreased in the Northeast and the Midwest. Total enrollments in master's programs increased in all regions, and total enrollment in doctoral programs increased in the Northeast but declined in all other regions. Graduations in doctoral programs increased in all regions.

Gender, race, and ethnicity statistics, which help identify the underrepresented populations, must also be addressed in order to direct specific retention strategies. The percentage of men in nursing education programs has increased during the past half-decade. Men comprise slightly less than 10 percent of all the enrollments in nursing schools (National League for Nursing, 1991). Approximately 9.5 percent of those enrolled in the generic baccalaureate programs and 5.2 percent of those in the RN programs, as reported by the American Association of Colleges of Nursing (1992), were male. The generic master's (master's for non-nursing college graduates) indicated 16.2 percent male. The greatest proportion of males is located in the West (6 percent) and the greatest number of male graduates is located in the South (National League for Nursing, 1991).

In 1989, the overall proportion of minority enrollments in nursing schools indicated African Americans comprised about 10 percent and Hispanics accounted for 3 percent of students enrolled in nursing schools. Enrollments of Asian Americans and American Indians are slightly lower in nursing schools than in colleges. Larger proportions of African American and Asian American students were enrolled in baccalaureate programs (12 percent and 3.1 percent). Hispanics had no differences in enrollment rates among different program types (National League for Nursing, 1991).

The American Association of Colleges of Nursing (1992) further indicated that American Indians or natives of Alaska represented up to 1.1 percent of the total number enrolled in baccalaureate and RN programs. Hispanics represented 2.9 percent of baccalaureate, 1.7 percent of master's, and 1.7 percent of doctoral students. African Americans represented 8.8 percent of those enrolled in generic baccalaureate and 7.4 percent of those enrolled in RN programs. Master's and doctoral program enrollments of African Americans diminished to 5.2 percent and 4.3 percent, respectively. Nonresident aliens represented less than 1 percent of those enrolled in baccalaureate, 1.1 percent of those in master's, and 2.6 percent of those in doctoral programs. Overall, there was little change in the proportion of racial and ethnic categories over a two-year (1990–1991) period. Although minorities are better represented in nursing than in other disciplines, there is a need to increase nursing programs' participation in recruitment and retention of underrepresented groups.

Review of research literature indicates that faculty should explore three major categories of retention strategies: (1) academic, (2) financial, and (3) support services. Retention strategies should be made available for all nursing students. Particular emphasis, however, should be placed on retention programs for the underrepresented groups, because of the higher attrition rates and lower enrollment figures of this particular population.

RESEARCH ON RETENTION STRATEGIES FOR MINORITY NURSING STUDENTS

Current studies relating specifically to minority nursing students include a variety of approaches for enhancement of retention strategies. Sutton and Claytor (1992) described the process of developing and implementing, for replication on other campuses, a comprehensive retention program for minority nursing students at a predominantly White, state, commuter school of nursing. The program is divided into four phases: (1) organization and mission, (2) available resources, (3) planning strategies, and (4) evaluation. Jones (1992) indicated the use of a developmental model for improving retention and graduation rates for African American students in nursing education.

Perceptions of African American women in a baccalaureate nursing program were examined by Quarry (1990). This descriptive study focused on factors that these women identified as hindering or promoting academic progress. The findings revealed that multiple barriers are perceived; the most significant barrier is academic workload. Participants identified the family as the most important support system.

Scott (1992) reported on a grant-funded program that included a study of why retention rates continue to be low, especially for minority and other high-risk students who were academically, economically, and/or socially disadvantaged. Specific problems were identified, and an educational specialist worked with the students individually or in groups. Referrals were made to other departments—reading and math laboratories, financial aid, and counseling.

Rogers (1990) indicated that minority students entering predominantly White colleges to major in nursing presented a unique challenge for faculty. These students are often considered to have been victims of long-term educational disadvantages and are, more than likely, academically underprepared for the rigor of college studies. The author identified academic and psychosocial factors that affect academic success. Retention strategies outlined for prenursing and nursing levels included: early identification of academic deficiencies and appropriate interventions; counseling for remedial work (developmental or enrichment); more aggressive advisement; and minority faculty recruitment, just to name a few.

The Getting Assistance In Nursing (GAIN) Project (Ormeaux & Redding, 1990) is a program to recruit and retain individuals from disadvantaged backgrounds. The effect of GAIN on a generic BSN program was reflected in an increase, among the graduates, of 12 percent of students who had been classified as disadvantaged. Retention methods according to the GAIN model, were made up of: (1) systematic screening to identify those at risk prior to major hurdles, and (2) strategies to increase chances for success. Assessment and intervention methods were described in detail. Enrollment in specified courses was indicated to achieve success in the program. In addition to implementing the GAIN model, student stipends were initiated. Eligibility status included full-time enrollment and financial, economical, and sociocultural disadvantaged status, as defined by the grant. Stipend recipients received individual academic counseling, peer tutoring in nursing courses, and personal counseling.

Anderson (1991) reported on results of nursing programs' survey of successful minority graduates in order to determine what they perceived to be most helpful in their success. Graduates identified six of ten retention factors as either highly or moderately influential. The two most influential factors were: (1) peer support and (2) faculty acceptance. Supportiveness of clinical personnel at hospitals, academic advisement or counseling, flexible scheduling, and individualized education options were identified as moderately influential in their retention. The factor that had the least effect was the presence of minority personnel, other than faculty and counselors. This finding suggests that role models may not play important parts in recruitment and retention of minority students at this particular campus. July (1988) suggested that the success and retention of African American students in baccalaureate nursing programs was related to the use of African American counselors and student housing.

Crawford and Olinger (1988) proposed several interventions to facilitate recruitment, retention, and graduation of culturally diverse students in baccalaureate programs:

1. Determine the level of institutional commitment to include culturally diverse backgrounds.
2. Increase faculty, staff, and administrative sensitivity to the needs of these students.
3. Increase cultural diversity content in the nursing curriculum.
4. Develop institutional support services to include academic advising, personal counseling services, remedial and developmental programs, and child care centers.
5. Increase financial resources and recruit minority faculty, staff, and administrators.
6. Provide extensive orientation programs.
7. Establish peer support groups and establish a multicultural center.
8. Develop linkages between colleges/universities and minority students in high school, middle school, and elementary schools.
9. Provide increased support to traditional African American institutions.

Specific attention has been given to ethnic minority nursing students for whom English is a second language. A rapidly growing number of nursing students are individuals whose primary language is not English. The English as a Second Language (ESL) group represents diverse racial and ethnic backgrounds. Phillips and Hartley

(1990) indicated that ESL students are found in greater numbers in nursing schools than in other baccalaureate programs. They contribute to the diversity of the profession but they experience language difficulties that may influence their academic achievement. Faculty need to be alert to bilingual students who may find reading assignments time-consuming and frustrating and who may need additional support to advance their English reading skills. Computer-assisted instruction (CAI) is a valuable tool for practice drills and critical thinking skills. Recording lectures and using visual displays during lectures can assist with deficient note-taking skills. Attention needs to be paid to clinical assignments, writing assignments, and learning styles of ESL students.

Memmer and Worth (1991) suggested that the most valid test predictors of successful completion of a generic nursing program are those that require effective use of English language skills. Their research, which described 30 retention approaches, addressed ways to assist ESL students to succeed in nursing programs. Although specific to 21 California nursing programs, many of these strategies may be generalized. Among the interventions described were: placement tests; remedial courses; terminology courses; career days; orientation programs; study skill workshops; writing workshops; family involvement; financial aid; mentor programs; ESL/minority faculty; flexible classload option; ratio of teacher–students in clinical lab; clinical lab grouping; peer tutorial assistance; and academic advisement.

RESEARCH AND INSTITUTIONAL CHARACTERISTICS

Cashion (1990) studied the retention of baccalaureate nursing students to determine whether there was a relationship between the predictor variables and students' decisions to persist in the program. Results indicated that the rate of retention at private colleges was 25 percent higher than for students at public schools. These results have retention implications for policy, curriculum development, and enrollment management strategies.

RESEARCH AND ECONOMIC/FINANCIAL CONSIDERATIONS

A major factor associated with nursing student retention and addressed within a multiple of studies is the financial or economic costs. To direct strategies in this area, costs of nursing education need to be presented. The American Association of Colleges of Nursing (1989) depicted several major findings:

1. An increased reliance on loans or self-funding of a nursing degree has resulted in a longer educational experience.
2. Registered nurse students returning for the baccalaureate rely heavily on personal savings and tuition reimbursement by their employers.
3. Students with a previous, non-nursing degree rely heavily on personal savings, spousal support, and work to fund their education.
4. At eight colleges surveyed, over 59 percent of the students reported that they would be employed during their education.

In addition to several other findings regarding the financial burden of a nursing education, this study suggested pursuit of important policy initiatives that can relieve the financial factor and facilitate retention of students.

Huch, Leonard, and Gutsch (1992) sought to develop a specification equation that could be used to predict retention in the academic area and the workplace. Once the results of personality testing were determined, the development of the equation could proceed. Such data, when gathered, can be used by an advisor to guide students. By identifying students who might contribute to the attrition rate, the resources of those students can be saved and directed to an area where the student may have a greater likelihood for success. Objective measures for student selection will assist with concentration on those students most likely to persist.

Retention strategies are generally found to incorporate multiple strategy approaches. Benda (1991) examined the relationship among the constructs in Tinto's model of college student retention. Components of results indicated that departed students were concerned with finances; thus, a retention strategy should be to secure efforts for funding for education of nursing. Demographic, pre-entry, academic institutional, social institutional, and commitment variables were also measured. Further results indicated that there were differences between retained and departed students. Retained freshmen scored higher on ACT subscores, two measures of high school grades, and high school class rank. Retained freshmen were more likely to choose a major other than nursing at the time of the ACT assessment, perceived more external control from institutional rules and regulations, and were more certain of their ability to pay for their education (Benda, 1989).

RESEARCH AND SPECIFIC RETENTION STRATEGIES

Additional studies have addressed specific retention strategies for nursing students. A variety of approaches with designated populations will be addressed in this section.

Cohen (1992) proposed consideration of status and power issues in nursing research, in theory, and at all levels of nursing education. Curricular reform and revision of nursing theories to emphasize the sociopolitical content of nursing will help change the socialization of student nurses. By stressing autonomy, independence, and confidence, recruitment and retention may be affected.

Backer (1989) emphasized the exploration of self-assessment of stress and coping as a stress management intervention with baccalaureate nursing students. The most significant finding of this project was that students are in need of focus on themselves as human beings. Faculty's role in responding to this need will help facilitate retention.

Academic emphasis was found in Campbell and Davis (1990), Glanville (1989), and Scott (1992). Scott (1992) stressed ranking problems of the disadvantaged student and providing the intervention relevant to the problems in class or clinical lab. Glanville (1989) explored an involvement program to increase retention of remedial prenursing students in a clinical nursing program. The results suggested that the involvement program successfully increased interest and retention among remedial prenursing students, and that, among students required to repeat remedial mathematics courses, those from the involvement program were more likely to persist. Campbell and Davis (1990) suggested that successful retention of at-risk nursing students is best accomplished through an organized system that addresses individual needs in the areas of academic, cognitive, and self-enhancement skills. The authors described the incentive, development, implementation, and value of the system, which can be adapted in any setting that has adequate human and material resources.

Henfling and Lowry (1990) demonstrated a creative response to concerns of retention of staff and students by developing an academically sound registered nurse education for a specific full-time employed population. This constituted a link between service and education in the provision of a convenient, low-cost, accessible education.

Several authors have indicated that nursing education needs to focus on program changes in order to retain students. Joel (1988) reported that students leaving the nursing major most frequently complained about rigidity of structure and little latitude for creativity and flexibility. Because student populations are not comprised of a high percentage of high school graduates, programs should be addressing the retention of transfer students, individuals making midlife and later life career changes, and students with special learning needs. Strategies include remedial help in basic skills, faculty-assisted seminars to support the sciences and nursing major courses, and tailored counseling services. An additional strength identified in a specific program was the maintenance of ties with alumni who mentored students and later helped graduates to access practice opportunities.

Hansen (1988) further stressed that the most important area to examine for student retention is the philosophy of the school of nursing toward its students and how that philosophy is transmitted to each student. Does each faculty member assist the student to succeed and graduate? Is an attitude of "Do it our way or not at all" still in existence? Is the program adaptable and flexible to needs of students with regard to class and clinical schedules? Hansen believes it is imperative that faculty examine requirements, schedules, and other policies in view of impediments that work against the student's succeeding. Among further strategies identified were: advisement and counseling; a student tutoring system; decision-making role modeling; and assistance with financial aid.

To further emphasize strategies faculty and administrators can develop for student retention, Thurber, Hollingsworth, Brown, and Whitaker (1989) presented an ideal model for enhancing student retention through effective, individualized, and consistent student advisement. Although the concept of a system of faculty advisement is not new, these authors viewed a successful adviser–advisee relationship as an essential part of the student's collegiate experience. The adviser role must be seen by faculty and administration as an important part of the productivity and evaluation criteria of the faculty. The model developed for this ideal school of nursing has several important principles. The faculty adviser is crucial to the student's initial orientation to the academic setting, and the role of the adviser is explained to each student. Beyond the initial establishment, every effort is made to keep the student with the same adviser throughout the program. There are specific instances, however, that indicate the benefit of changing advisers. It is also understood that the adviser role will change as the student advances through the program. It is felt that a comprehensive, individualized advising program is one way to increase satisfaction, which in turn increases retention in the nursing major.

Courage and Godbey (1992) described the academic services and policies of a retention program for nursing students. Central to this program is the integration of students into the life of the institution. Services include orientation, tutoring, advisement, progress monitoring, achievement awards, and stress management. The critical elements identified for the program are: nursing faculty commitment to the retention of students; faculty commitment to the program for retention; integration of students into the college of nursing upon student entry; and immediate individualized intervention. Policies addressed to support this program include those related to readmission, individual study, and course repetition. Specific types of programs for nursing student retention in nursing education can be found in current literature as well. Several of these strategies focus on the needs of specified underrepresented populations. Phillips and Hartley (1990) addressed language difficulties of nursing students for whom English is a second language and identified use of preferential learning styles that need to be considered for curriculum development and classroom strategies. Memmer and Worth (1991) described retention approaches for ESL students as well.

Remedial mathematics programs have been addressed in many multifaceted approaches to retention. The purpose of Glanville's (1989) study was to develop an exploratory involvement program to address both the use of nursing language and nursing examples in a remedial mathematics program for prenursing students. The author also looked at the students' involvement in selected clinical nursing co-curricular activities to determine whether both of these aspects affect the students' interest and persistence in the remedial mathematics course and retention in the college. As previously discussed, an involvement program increased interest and retention.

Cook and Thurmand (1989) identified the development and implementation of nursing courses, curriculum design, program evaluation, and program specifics of a nursing Student Educational Enrichment Program (SEEP). This program was developed for minority nursing students in order to improve retention rates of minorities enrolled.

DISCUSSION AND RECOMMENDATIONS

Many strategies are available for retention of nursing students. Table 1 provides an overview of several studies on student nurse retention strategies. These strategies should be tailored to the educational program's recruitment pool (Joel, 1988). Faculty will need to be committed to any given program. Policies and procedures effectively utilized for traditional education need to be modified to meet the needs of today's students.

Academic services, which may include flexible scheduling of classes or clinical lab times, summer sessions, night and weekend alternatives, advanced placement, challenge options, and assessment of life experience for credit will facilitate progress and reinforce an expression of interest in the student (Joel, 1988). Academic advisement programs, tutorial and mentoring services, and individualized or group sessions all need to be explored. Remedial skills assistance for all students, especially the underrepresented populations, should be implemented as indicated. Innovative teaching strategies such as CAI and other critical thinking approaches need to be studied. Faculty and administration must recognize that some radical changes may be indicated in order to improve the academic services provided to today's students.

Financial aid implications for students who remain in nursing have become even more critical today, with cuts in higher education and scholarship programs. Additional research needs to be conducted to provide a basis for outlining costs students incur in pursuit of nursing degrees. To get a true picture of the actual expenses incurred, *total* degree costs should be analyzed: education costs, living expenses, net income foregone, and loan payback costs. Several nursing students have considerable difficulty securing financial aid, which detracts from both recruitment and retention of students. There appears to be a large amount of unmet financial need as well as a high total indebtedness upon graduation (American Association of Colleges of Nursing, 1989). Strategies need to be further developed to provide additional models and methods of obtaining and examining costs. Faculty and university administration, along with health care agencies, need to work diligently to develop effective methods to resolve financial restrictions that are hindering the educational advancement of nursing students.

Access to and availability of support services are of primary concern to students. Families have been cited as one of the most positive supports (Quarry, 1990). Faculty advisement and mentorships are

Table 1. Summary of Studies on Student Nurse Retention/Strategies

Author/Date	Subject of Research	Variable/Instruments	Sample	Research/Design Statistics	Findings
Anderson, 1991	A survey of successful minority graduates to determine their perception of what was most helpful to their success in the nursing programs.	Survey that replicates one by Quintilian.	44 minority graduates from licensed vocational and associate degree nursing programs on the West Coast.	Descriptive.	Graduates did not identify any factors as highly influential to their recruitment. They did identify 6 of 10 retention factors as highly or moderately influential. Most influential factors were peer supportiveness and faculty acceptance and helpfulness. The factor that had the least effect on retention of minority students was the presence of minority personnel, other than faculty and counselors.
Backer, 1989	Exploration of utilization of self-assessment of stress and coping as stress management intervention with baccalaureate nursing students.	Interview, an evaluative coping scale, and an evaluation form.	55 students enrolled in their first clinical course in nursing in an urban northeastern university.	Quasi-experimental.	Results did not indicate significant increases in frequency and use of coping strategies pre- and postintervention. There were shifts of coping methods used over the semester.
Benda, 1989	An investigation of demographic, pre-entry, academic institutional, social institutional, and commitment variables associated with retention.	ACT assessments prior to college entry and a 104-item questionnaire.	188 freshmen, 141 sophomores, and 23 junior baccalaureate nursing students.	Descriptive survey, *t*-tests and chi-square analysis, ANOVA.	Retained freshmen scored higher than departed students on ACT subscores, mathematics, and composite on two measures of high school grades and high school class rank. Retained

					freshmen were also more likely to choose a major other than nursing at the time of ACT assessment, perceived more external control from institutional rules and regulations, and were more certain of their ability to pay for their education. The variables were examined across academic classes.
Bruyere, 1991	Addressing the needs of "high-risk" students who do not have adequate academic prerequisites.	Questionnaire.	Single parents, aboriginal Canadians, and immigrants in a nursing program in Canada.	Descriptive.	Findings of questionnaire revealed that native students thought they were seen as passive, shy, noninterfering, and reserved. A variety of responses emphasized that it is imperative in nursing to recognize that demand for personal and academic growth is greater for minority students.
Campbell & Davis, 1990	Development of Enrichment for Academic Success (EAS) system.	Analysis of data that identified characteristics of students at risk of not successfully completing the nursing program and those at risk of being unsuccessful as first-time writers	320 students enrolled in nursing program in the South.	Descriptive analysis of demographics of the survey; summary of factors.	Based on the assessment information, a retention plan, Enrichment for Academic Success (EAS), was implemented. The effectiveness of EAS was determined by formative and summative data. Overall retention rate of the program participants was 95.4 percent.

Table 1. *(Continued)*

Author/ Date	Subject of Research	Variable/ Instruments	Sample	Research/Design Statistics	Findings
		of the NCLEX-RN. Survey to identify factors students believed contributed to or hindered progression.			
Cashion, 1990	Exploration of student and institutional characteristics to determine whether there is a relationship between predictor variables and a student's decision to remain in a program.	Eight variable sets added into a regression equation: (1) student background, (2) education aspiration, (3) personality and value, (4) institutional, (5) transfer, (6) financial aid, (7) interpersonal interaction, and (8) college achievement.	279 women.	Longitudinal survey; descriptive; multilinear regression.	Three variables were significant: (1) institutional control, (2) satisfaction with the institution of initial entry, and (3) the number of institutions attended. Retention rate of students at private colleges was 25 percent higher than that of students at public schools. Transferring to a second college decreased persistence by 15 percent. Being satisfied with initial college increased persistence by 34 percent.
Cook & Thurmand, 1989	Development, implementation, and evaluation of a nursing Student Educational Enrichment Program (SEEP) for minority nursing students.	27-item evaluation tool with a 5-point Likert-type scale; evaluation of grades.	6 nursing students selected; only 4 enrolled in summer nursing program.	Descriptive survey.	Evaluation of non-nursing courses indicated a positive response to the value and usefulness of support courses. Evaluation of nursing courses indicated benefits of SEEP program.

					Comments and evaluations were considered helpful in planning future programs.
Glanville, 1989	The development of an explanatory involvement program to address whether both the use of nursing language and nursing examples in a remedial math program and involvement in clinical nursing affects prenursing students' interest and persistence in the math course and retention in college.	Involvement in a special remedial course with specific factors.	Experimental group: 52 prenursing students requiring remedial math; control group: 44 prenursing students in a traditional remedial math program.	Descriptive.	Involvement program successfully increased interest and retention among remedial prenursing students.
Huch, Leonard, & Gutsch, 1992	The development of a specification equation that could be used to predict retention of nursing students in a selected program of study.	Form A of the 16PF.	151 nursing majors at a southern public university.	Two-step design; longitudinal; univariate F test on each of the 16PF factors; discriminant analysis.	Results identified personality traits (PT) that relate to needs of students and help formulate advisement. PT data also assist advisers to know students and students to know themselves.
July, 1988	Identification of model practices that enhance marketing, recruitment, and retention of African American students in baccalaureate nursing programs and in nursing.	Investigator-developed questionnaire.	23 nursing schools.	Descriptive.	Recruitment/retention of African American nursing students needs new creative approaches. Enrollment of this population in nursing schools has not changed over the past 10 years.
Memmer & Worth, 1991	Approaches used in all of California's 21 generic baccalaureate nursing programs to retain ESL students.	Telephone interview, structured questionnaire.	21 program directors or their designees.	Descriptive.	Thirty retention approaches are described. Of the 21 programs, 5 had ESL retention rates of 93 percent of students.

Table 1. (*Continued*)

Author/ Date	Subject of Research	Variable/ Instruments	Sample	Research/Design Statistics	Findings
Quarry, 1990	Identification of the kinds of support systems successful African American adults perceive as having contributed to academic progress and retention.	Semistructured interview, closed-ended demographic questionnaire.	25 women in junior year of an urban public institution.	Descriptive.	Study participants perceived multiple barriers to their academic progress—most significantly, the academic workload. The family was identified as a significant support system.
Rosenfeld, 1988	Statistical measurement of retention with factors that contribute to retention problem of nursing education programs—annual survey.	Questionnaire.	235 diploma, 364 BSN, 675 ADN programs	Descriptive.	Diploma programs have lower retention rates. Nursing has higher retention rates than general retention rates in colleges. Students have difficulty with required courses, personal problems/family obligations, financial difficulties, and inability to find jobs.
Woodtli, Hazzard, & Rusch, 1988	Joint development and support, by an educational institution and a nursing service agency, of a student internship program.	Program evaluation questionnaires.	19 students and nurse preceptors.	Pilot study of senior student nursing internship—classroom work, work study, and preceptorship.	Student internship program in the final semester of the senior year had positive outcomes in areas of program satisfaction, institutional collaboration, recruitment cost, and retention rates.

suggested to strengthen the development of the nursing student's image, as well as to function as reliable sources who provide access to referral services. University counseling, advisement, and other specialized programs need to be more vigorously incorporated, even with the financial restraints, to help provide the support needed.

Crawford and Olinger (1988) stressed that, although many avenues available may require financial support, others simply need a more positive philosophical approach. Today, colleges, universities, and individuals must be willing to do their part in the all-important endeavor to retain every nursing student.

REFERENCES

American Association of Colleges of Nursing. (1989). *The economic investment in nursing education: Student institutional and clinical perspectives.* Washington, DC: The Association.

American Association of Colleges of Nursing. (1992). *Enrollment and graduations in baccalaureate and graduate programs in nursing.* Washington, DC: The Association.

Anderson, J. (1991). Nursing students: Minority recruitment and retention. *Nurse Educator, 16*(5), 38–39.

Backer, B. A. (1989). *Utilization of assessment as an intervention in nursing student stress: An exploratory project.* Unpublished doctoral dissertation, City University of New York, New York.

Benda, E. J. (1989). *A study of variables associated with retention of baccalaureate nursing students.* Unpublished doctoral dissertation, The University of Iowa,

Benda, E. J. (1991). The relationship among variables in Tinto's conceptual model and attrition of bachelor's degree nursing students. *Journal of Professional Nursing, 7*(1), 16–24.

Bliesmer, M., & Eggenberger, S. (1989). Strategies for recruiting nursing students. *Nurse Educator, 14*(2), 17–20.

Bruyere, J. (199). Personal growth and the minority student. *Journal of Nursing Education, 30*(6), 278–279.

Campbell, A. R., & Davis, S. M. (1990). Enrichment for academic success: Helping at-risk students. *Nurse Educator, 15*(6), 33–37.

Cashion, C. F. (1990). *Retention of baccalaureate nursing students.* Unpublished doctoral dissertation, Syracuse University, Syracuse, NY.

Cohen, L. B. (1992). Power and change in health care: Challenge for nursing. *Journal of Nursing Education, 31*(3), 113–116.

Cook, P. R., & Thurmand, V. (1989). Summer program for prematriculating nursing students. *Journal of Black Nurses' Association, 3*(1), 54–63.

Courage, M. M., & Godbey, K. L. (1992). Student retention: Policies and services to enhance persistence to graduation. *Nurse Educator, 17*(2), 29–32.

Crawford, L. A., & Olinger, B. H. (1988). Recruitment and retention of nursing students from diverse cultural backgrounds. *Journal of Nursing Educator, 27*(8), 379–381.

Fralic, M. F. (1988). Response to retention strategies in nursing education panel. In *Nursing shortage: Strategies for nursing practice and education* (pp. 113–114). Report of the National Invitational Workshop. Washington, DC: U.S. Department of Health and Human Services, Publications Division.

Glanville, W. B. (1989). *An involvement program to increase retention of remedial prenursing students in a clinical nursing program: Implications for public urban community college educators.* Unpublished doctoral dissertation, Teachers College, Columbia University, New York.

Hansen, G. (1988). Student retention in associate degree nursing education. In *Nursing shortage: Strategies for nursing practice and education.* Report of the National Invitational Workshop. Washington, DC: U.S. Department of Health and Human Services, Publications Division.

Henfling, P. A., & Lowry, L. W. (1990). Nursing shortage: Catalyst for administrative/educational partnership. *Journal of Nursing Staff Development, 6*(3), 121–125.

Heydman, A. (1991). Retention/attrition of nursing students: Emphasis on disadvantaged and minority students. In P. A. Baj & G. M. Clayton (Eds.), *Review of research in nursing education* (pp. 1–29). New York: National League for Nursing.

Huch, M. H., Leonard, R. L., & Gutsch, K. U. (1992). Nursing education: Developing specification equations for selection and retention. *Journal of Professional Nursing, 8*(3), 170–175.

Joel, L. A. (1988). Retention strategies in nursing education. In *Nursing shortage: Strategies for nursing practice and education.* Report of the National Invitational Workshop. Washington, DC: U.S. Department of Health and Human Services, Publications Division.

Jones, S. H. (1992). Improving retention and graduation rates for Black students in nursing education: A developmental model. *Nursing Outlook, 40*(2), 78–85.

July, F. M. (1988). *Recruitment and retention of Black students in baccalaureate nursing programs: An application of the marketing process.* Unpublished doctoral dissertation, Georgia State University College of Education,

Kleffel, D. (1988). Response to retention strategies in nursing education panel. In *Nursing shortage for nursing practice and education* (pp. 115–116). Report of the National Invitational Workshop. Washington, DC: U.S. Department of Health and Human Services, Publications Division.

Memmer, M. K., & Worth, C. C. (1991). Retention of English as a second language (ESL) students: Approaches used by California's 21 generic baccalaureate nursing programs. *Journal of Nursing Education, 30*(9), 389–396.

National League for Nursing. (1991). *Nursing Data Review 1991.* New York: National League for Nursing Press.

Ormeaux, S. D., & Redding, E. A. (1990). GAIN: A successful recruitment and retention program for disadvantaged students. *Journal of Nursing Education, 29*(9), 412–414.

Phillips, S., & Hartley, J. (1990). Teaching students for whom English is a second language. *Nurse Educator, 15*(5), 29–32.

Quarry, N. E. (1990). Perceptions of Black adults about their academic progress in a baccalaureate nursing program. *Journal of National Black Nurses' Association, 4*(2), 28–36.

Rodgers, S. G. (1990). Retention of minority nursing students on predominantly White campuses. *Nursing Educator, 15*(5), 36–39.

Rosenfeld, P. (1988). Measuring student retention: A national analysis. *Nursing and Health Care, 9*(4), 199–200.

Santovec, M. L. (Ed.). (1990). *Building diversity: Recruitment and retention in the 90's.* Wisconsin: Magna Publications.

Scott, S. (1992). Educational specialist: Grant-funded instructional and clinical support for minority and high-risk nursing students. *Journal of Nursing Education, 31*(1), 40–41.

Sutton, L., & Claytor, K. (1992). Enhancing minority nursing student success through a comprehensive retention program. *Association of Black Nursing Faculty Journal, 3*(2), 31–37.

Thurber, F. H., Hollingsworth, A., Brown, L., & Whitaker, S. (1989). The faculty advisor role: An imperative for student retention. *Nurse Educator, 14*(3), 27–29.

Williams, M. T. (1988). Policies and procedures for scheduling student nurses. *Journal of Nursing Administration, 18*(9), 32–37.

Woodtli, A., Hazzard, M. E., & Rusch, S. (1988). Senior internship: A strategy for recruitment, retention, and collaboration. *Nursing Connections, 1*(3), 37–50.

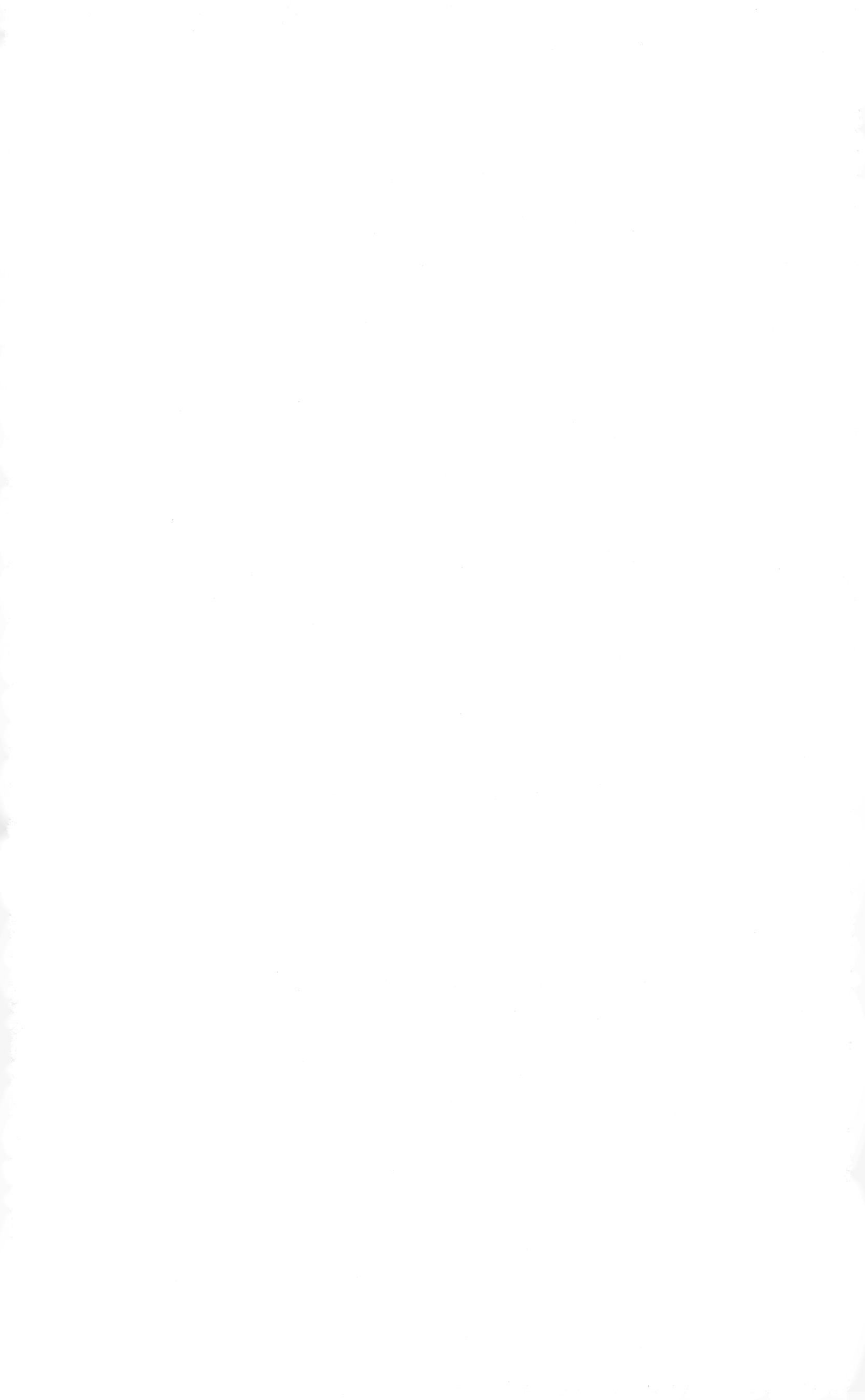